The Ketogenic Reset:

The ultimate beginner's guide to the perfect keto diet, simple and with clarity for women and men.

Josh Lee

2

© COPYRIGHT 2019 - ALL RIGHTS RESERVED.

TABLE OF CONTENTS

Introduction

Whether you have found your way here because you are looking to lose weight, are trying to manage a medical condition, or simply want to live a healthier lifestyle, you have come to the right place. The diet and fitness world can be scary and intimidating if you do not know what to look for, and if you aren't sure that your sources are trustworthy, you might be getting the wrong information. The ketogenic reset is not just about learning to cook healthier recipes. A ketogenic reset diet aims to reinvent your lifestyle with a stronger focus on eating natural, whole ingredients, with lower amounts of carbohydrates and higher concentrations of healthy fats. While carbohydrates from natural sources in regulated amounts are not necessarily bad for you, all carbs are sugars, and sugars of any type are unhealthy if you over-eat. A keto reset removes most of the carbohydrate content from your diet in order to fuel one of your body's lesser-known mechanisms of energy harvesting: fat breakdown. When you eat glucose, your body likes to metabolize it first before fat, because glucose is easier for us to digest. A ketogenic diet supplies your body with only healthy fats and no glucose, which means that there are no unhealthy sugars present for you to absorb. Instead, our bodies are forced to digest and use the energy we can get from fatty acid particles. If you are one of the many people who had no idea that fat could be *healthy*, the keto diet is the perfect way to introduce yourself to the world of nutritious fats and oils. When we eat these healthy fats and oils that are found in nature, we digest their broken-down pieces as fatty acids. Fatty acids provide our bodies with almost three times the amount of energy that one glucose molecule can, which is why the keto diet slowly convinces your body to switch. Although fatty acids do create a backlog of harmful acid build-up that glucose does *not*, there are still plenty of ways to manage a slight acidic concentration in your blood. The magic behind the ketogenic reset comes in the smaller digestive details. Instead of digesting too much glucose and storing it like sugar in our fat cells, the keto diet forces your body to digest fat, which has to be purged as an acid instead and will not end up increasing our weight. There are plenty of medical considerations and health concerns that coincide with the keto diet, and as with any new eating pattern, you should always consult with your doctor first. However, the ketogenic diet is not a fad, and it certainly is not a tea that you can drink to drop pounds. The ketogenic reset is a scientific and biologically natural mechanism shift that allows your body to do what it was naturally designed to do, and it is only an added benefit that you will lose weight. The keto diet is a highly detailed road map to give you the results you want without putting you through the rigorous diet standards that you do not need. On a keto diet, you will eat until you are full, snack, whenever you like and indulge in some of the most decadent diet meals you didn't think, were possible. It is time we all took a hard look at what we're putting in our bodies, and start to change our nutrition from the inside out. If you know what benefits you are giving your body before you even sit down to eat, you will be able to sustain a healthy, thin weight, for a longer time, with *fewer* health concerns than many people today. A ketogenic reset does not just offer a "refresh" button for your body. When you eat on a keto diet, you will be able to control things other diets only dream of: you can lower your blood pressure, lower your blood sugar, decrease your bad cholesterol and raise your good cholesterol, control the symptoms of your depression and anxiety, and even help abate the frequency of seizures associated with epilepsy. So many modern diseases can benefit from a low carbohydrate diet, and it is about time you showed your body the care and knowledge in fueling it the food that you deserve. If you are ready to jump in to a ketogenic reset diet and find out what science, and your body, can do for your weight loss potential, it is time to get you started. Once you have worked your way through the following chapter guides, you will have all the tools you need to prepare your body, thoughtfully begin a keto diet, and manage your health throughout to ensure safety and results. The health and nutrition world is always changing, but the keto diet itself is known for being one of the most open and flexible diets to learning, interpreting, and advancing the guidelines of a healthy keto lifestyle. If you or a friend try the ketogenic diet and want to share your experience, or you find that the information in this guide was helpful, please feel free to leave a comment in the review section. Joining in with the keto community is one of the most valuable benefits of a ketogenic reset. Our bodies are all different, and you might be able to learn a few things from your keto peers that could help you succeed. Plus, the more keto friends you make, the more hands you will have to help you meal prep on weekends. Fitness, and especially the ketogenic reset, is all about living your best life without changing the habits you already love. Get ready, and get hungry, because it is time to begin your ketogenic reset and help your body get back on track!

The Science of Weight Loss

Weight loss is one of the most controversial and confusing aspects of modern life. From herbal tea cleanses that prohibit solid foods to eating *only* fat, there are far too many techniques and theories. The human body is affected by hundreds of factors that can either support our health or contribute to chronic illness. Oftentimes the food groups and types of nutrition that we choose are not as healthy as we think, and even vegetarians and vegans can end up with high blood pressure, high cholesterol levels, and nutrient deficiency. But there are people who manage to eat healthy, sustainable diets without gaining weight – and without subscribing to intense workout regimes. The important crossover between fitness and science comes in understanding your body's relationship to fuel. If you know what type of fuel is best for achieving your weight loss goals, you will already be predisposed to lose more weight. Once you combine a targeted diet with an exercise routine that fits your lifestyle, you will lose weight. Losing weight without understanding your body's mechanisms is just the same as guessing and checking, but when it comes to science and fitness, you know that nothing is instant. So why would you choose to guess and check a weight loss plan that you are not positive can produce the results you want? Determining what sustains your body and controlling your nutrition from the start will allow you to help your body clear out toxins and impurities first. This will be inevitably accompanied by weight loss "without even trying" before you begin to really fuel yourself for daily activity. The theory behind this style of dieting is not a theory at all – it is real science, and that could be why so many people have yet to try, or even hear about, the ketogenic diet. Based on the natural science of your body's metabolic mechanisms, the keto diet is not a detox or a juice cleanse – it is a lifestyle change that will re-wire your body for natural and sustainable weight loss. Most people can't even pinpoint where their weight loss or dieting is going wrong, and that's most likely because they are unfamiliar with their bodies. Part of the magic of a ketogenic reset is that your new lifestyle teaches you invaluable knowledge about what your nutrition body needs and how it is going to use it. Even small things like your metabolism might not be what you think it is, and if you find yourself wondering, it's probably one of the many factors that might be causing you to pack on pounds. Luckily, keto begins and ends with your metabolism, so it's a great place to get started. Your body's metabolism is defined as the sum of all the processes that your systems undergo on a daily basis to sustain life. Many people incorrectly think that their metabolism is simply "how well their body burns fat" instead of "how effectively their body is being fueled to live". If you change your mindset like you did when you thought about crash diets, eating food groups that effectively fuel your body for the long-term will immediately help you lose weight. And that's even *before* you implement a ketogenic diet. But now that you understand how the keto diets aim to fuel your body; let's talk more in-depth about metabolism, and the secret metabolic mechanism that your body has to help you lose weight while you're eating keto.

Re-Wiring Your Metabolism on Keto

Glucose Metabolism and Too Much Sugar

The human body contains a hierarchy of processes that we use to digest food, and although we would prefer to digest glucose only, our body comes with a hierarchy just in case all the conditions for digestion aren't met. The process by which our bodies take energy from digested food is called cellular respiration, and it involves more than a few steps.

However, our cells can perform respiration in multiple different restricted environments in case we need energy but are struggling elsewhere. A great example of this is during an intense workout, or when our bodies are lacking certain nutrients that help facilitate digestion. Regularly, our bodies like to digest glucose as a fuel source the most, because the process of digesting and harvesting sugar is easiest. Glucose is often referred to as a "simple sugar", yes, but it isn't the sugars you are used to. Glucose is technically a monosaccharide, which is one of our body's favorite types of sustenance. Glucose, a healthy monosaccharide, and fructose and lactose, unhealthy disaccharides, are the three main types of sugars that our body can convert into energy. Glucose is the most necessary to our diets, and it can be found in almost anything – it is the main ingredient in almost all carbohydrates. From fruits and vegetables to grains, yeasts, and seeds, our bodies use the glucose in carbs as their main fuel source because it can be digested and converted into energy without oxygen. Cellular respiration can take place either aerobically, which means with oxygen, or anaerobically, which means without oxygen. When you are breathing hard at the gym, it is likely that your muscles are not getting enough oxygen to produce the amount of energy they need to output. If oxygen is not present, our bodies can focus on one of the mechanisms of glucose-driven cellular respiration and change it. This change allows us to harvest energy during a tough workout with minimal damage, although it is not our ideal way of getting energy. However, there is a catch to digesting glucose as our main fuel source, and it's a catch that will definitely prevent you from achieving a healthy weight. Glucose is fine in portioned doses, but think about what happens when you eat too much sugar. Whether it's too many fruits or too many processed sugars, an excess of glucose will cause you to pack on stored sugar that your body is unlikely to use. Changing your fuel source doesn't just keep unhealthy amounts of fat out of your diet, though; it also keeps unhealthy fat off of your waistline. So how does the keto diet fuel your body if you aren't eating your biologically preferred fuel source? Just because glucose metabolism is preferred doesn't mean it is the best possible mechanism for your body to use - and just because our cells need glucose doesn't mean it is the healthiest thing for us. The ketogenic diet shifts your body from metabolizing carbohydrates to metabolizing healthy fats, which is a whole new method of cellular respiration that can have an incredible and instant impact on your health, while also helping you sustain healthy habits for years to come.

Why Ketogenic Diets Choose to Metabolize Fat

Metabolizing fat instead of glucose creates a bi-product that your body will not store as sugar or fat that is similar to the bi-product you create during cellular respiration – and this bi-product is a weight-loss powerhouse. When you're working out, your body converts part of your broken down glucose molecules into a form of acid, called lactic acid. While you might have heard of lactic acid before, it is not actually the cause of sore muscles after an intense sweat session. Lactic acid is simply an in-between molecule that your body creates in order to break down energy without oxygen. When you fuel your body with healthy fats only (yes, fats can be healthy, but do not worry – we will cover that more in Chapter Two) you create a similar bi-product that is also an acid. Sometimes called "keto acid", this substance contains molecules called ketone bodies that are made up of acids and other small chemical groups. Luckily, this bi-product does not get stored in your body if you consume too much fatty food, unlike glucose. Instead, there are a few ways that your body handles this build-up of ketone bodies during the keto diet. You will use a few guidelines and tips to help purge your body of this acid, but overall, its effects on your health can be easily managed. Modifying your fuel source to consist of mostly fats has more than a few health benefits, mainly because you will not be packing on extra unhealthy fat is delicate places. Low levels of consumed glucose have been proven to help lower your blood pressure and decrease your blood sugar levels, particularly as these two conditions relate to atherosclerosis or the swelling of over-taxed heart muscles. Obviously, lower levels of glucose eaten mean lower levels of glucose in your blood, but this can be key medical information for many individuals diagnosed with Type 2 diabetes. Although Chapter Three will talk further about the health benefits and risks of eating a keto diet, the up-front benefits are highly logical and scientifically proven. The keto diet itself was developed similarly to the Atkin's diet to control outside triggers for autoimmune diseases like Parkinson's disease, chronic epilepsy, arthritis, and even Alzheimer's. Since its beginnings, however, a low carbohydrate, the high fat keto diet has also been proven to help with insomnia and sleep disorders, chronically low energy levels, depression, and anxiety. Besides these numerous medical benefits, diets low in carbohydrates also tend to keep you fuller for longer, helping to control your appetite and stabilize your eating patterns. But this style of appetite suppression is not actually dangerous, and in fact, it is something that your body is probably doing incorrectly in the first place. To understand more about how the keto diet controls your appetite and suppresses cravings, we need to talk about insulin.

Decreased Appetite and the Function of Insulin

One of the easiest ways to understand how the keto diet works is to examine weight loss only as it relates to your body's insulin levels. Insulin, which we've touched on briefly before, does tens of crucial things throughout the body that are vital to our daily function. However, in the case of appetite, your insulin has little control. Produced and released by the pancreas, insulin levels spike whenever there is lots of glucose present in your system. Carbohydrate-rich foods that are packed with sugars will cause an immediate rise in your blood sugar levels, which will trigger your pancreas to flood your bloodstream with insulin. Once the insulin arrives, however, there is not any glucose left, and the result is an immediate hunger right after you've just eaten a huge meal. The root of the problem here is not your insulin, or your pancreas – it is your diet. If you eat more fats and proteins, your body learns to adjust to food that takes longer to digest, and offers fewer sugary carbohydrates. Longer digestion also means feeling fuller for longer, which means a keto diet eliminates two types of appetite confusion, instead of just one. The fats and proteins that you will be eating on a ketogenic diet will raise your blood sugar levels slowly and safely, which will prevent that flood of insulin from your pancreas. On a keto diet, you will not experience as many distinctive "hunger pangs" as you normally would if you were consuming carbohydrates. But that is not all the insulin has to offer you on a ketogenic diet. Insulin is also the chemical that controls fat storage in our muscles, liver, and fat cells. High quantities of insulin in the bloodstream paired with a diet high in carbohydrates means you will be storing more fat than you need, and more fat than your body is telling you to. When you stick to eating a minimal carbohydrate diet that tends to keep your blood sugar low, and your carbohydrate content contained, you will find that you will not store as much unwanted fat, and can lose weight all the while you feel full and satisfied.

Your Body on the Keto Diet

What Does a Ketogenic Reset Taste Like?

The ketogenic diet, as you have surely now gathered, is focused on fueling your body with healthy fats only while drastically reducing your amount of daily carbohydrates. While you might think that this only applies to carbohydrates like grains, starches, and fibers, the ketogenic diet is notoriously strict on sugars. When you are eating on a keto diet, even the carbohydrates found in high-fiber, starchy vegetables and plants are off-limits. If you are not a vegetarian or vegan, you should also keep in mind that there is plenty of "lactose", or milk sugar, found in animal-derivative dairy products like cheese, yogurt, and cream. The interesting quirk about re-wiring your body for a ketogenic metabolism is that you are using a lesser metabolic method that your biology is not used to – which means your system will constantly be trying to return to digesting glucose. Any introduction of sugar into your bloodstream, whether it is healthy or not, might prevent your body from migrating to a full-time state of ketosis. We will define ketosis in greater detail in Chapter Four, but for now, you can just think of it as "the state of digesting only fat". For this reason, a ketogenic diet focuses on eating only specific subsets of your regular healthy food groups and controlling your portions in order to control your weight loss. While this sounds easy enough, you also have to make sure that you are controlling what your portions are made of. This is one of a few difficult quirks that come along with eating a strict keto diet, but we will go over these finer details during the "Frequently Asked Questions" section. In the meantime, let's take a closer look at what types of foods you will be able to eat on the keto diet, and which sorts of processed, unhealthy ingredients you are going to want to avoid.

Choosing Healthy Fats

Learning about the keto diet is an interesting journey if you are not familiar with healthy fats and sugars – particularly healthy fats. Most of us have been conditioned to believe that if it has "fat" in the name, it is not a nutritional choice. Much like the definition of metabolism, the concept of healthy and unhealthy fat has become so distorted by the fitness community that most people miss out on some of the most delicious, and beneficial, natural ingredients. For years, no one ate avocados because they are packed full of whole fats and oils – things that scientists thought were bad for us. Come to find out, fats that occur in nature, particularly from whole sources like vegetables, nuts, seeds, and oils provide our bodies with healthy monounsaturated fats. Monounsaturated fats are fats that have not undergone the tempering process of hydrogenation, in which the food packaging industry chemically alters the structure of a fat molecule so that it will last longer on the shelves. These fats, also known as saturated or trans fats, are no longer the healthy and natural molecules that they were before they were altered. Monounsaturated healthy fats function to lower our body's levels of bad cholesterol and raise our levels of good cholesterol. If you were not aware that cholesterol is not just one number, do not worry – plenty of people think that "cholesterol" is a catch-all term. In reality, cholesterol is a lipid-like molecule that helps our bodies with just about everything from neural function and brain regeneration to digestion and hormone production. Good cholesterol, known scientifically as high-density lipoprotein (HDL), is found in all healthy monounsaturated fats. The keto diet, while focused on fueling your body with only fat, is not focused on fueling your body with unhealthy fats. When it comes to choosing what to eat on a keto diet, it is imperative to make sure that you aren't getting your fats from saturated sources.

Low-density lipoproteins (LDLs) are the bad molecules of cholesterol that will force your heart into a state of constant over-working, not to mention stunt your overall weight loss and most likely make you gain pounds instead of losing them. Picking healthy fats means the difference between a whole new you, and a guess-and-check diet that doesn't leave you healthier, skinnier, or satisfied.

Ketogenic Ingredients and Recipes

Ketogenic recipes are definitely not what you are probably thinking, and that is a delicious thing. Unlike most diet meals and entrees, a keto diet tends to be packed with filling and delicious items that are high in healthy fats, and therefore not the stereotypical "diet foods". When you are eating keto-style, it is crucial that your "ketogenic food pyramid" is focused on healthy oils and fats first before moving on to non-red meats, eggs, and fish. Although you are still allowed to eat red, yellow, and orange starchy vegetables with higher carbohydrate contents, they come only after you have satisfied your diet with those antioxidant-packed dark green veggies. Nuts and small berries that are dark red or dark blue in color (excluding cherries, which are the fruits with the highest sugar content) come at the very end of the pyramid, but there is a little bit of wiggle room in between for full-fat dairy products like whole mozzarella cheese and full-fat coconut milk. You might be surprised to find out that a ketogenic diet is often packed full of fatty, sweet desserts because there are so many delicious ways to use natural fats and oils in baking sweet treats. While you will not be able to eat things like grainy pasta, rice, or almost any potatoes, keto diet experts have made it incredibly easy to substitute in delicious replacements for these foods. Zucchini or carrot homemade spaghetti noodles taste even better than regular pasta when they are cooked with parmesan cheese and warm marinara sauce. Quinoa tastes just as good as any brown rice and takes one-fifth the amount of time to cook without a pressure cooker. Plenty of chickpea mashes, and squash dishes make great substitutions for creamy potato sides, and if you have not ever tired cauliflower imposter chicken wings, it is about time you did. Many keto recipes are easy to cook because they do not require too many ingredients – the value of a delicious keto recipe is in the spice profile. You will want to make sure that you have a wide array of Italian, Greek, Middle-Eastern, Spanish, Indian, and Asian seasonings on-hand while you are cooking ketogenic meals. It is not a big mystery why plenty of these regions boast thinner and healthier populations: they've been eating keto-style for quite a while, cooking with monounsaturated fats and oils, and relying on whole fats instead of carbohydrates. However, if you aren't familiar with some of these cuisines right away, do not worry. The keto diet has plenty of easy staple meals for each time of day that will keep you satisfied and interested without running you back and forth from the grocery store. Here are a few keto recipe ideas for creative inspiration while you are trying to figure out which ingredients will fit best into your keto reset.

Tasty Keto Entrees for Each Meal

Keto Breakfast Ideas

The keto diet might be one of the only weight loss programs that allow you to eat a fried egg breakfast sandwich with two turkey sausage patties instead of carbohydrate-packed bread. While not all keto meals contain meat, eggs and turkey are both protein-filled food that work well to full you first thing in the morning and keep you satisfied until lunchtime. The key to making healthy hot breakfast dishes while you are eating a keto diet is to switch out your cooking ingredients. Instead of using cow butter or margarine, try high-fat olive oil or a delicious avocado oil at a low roasting temperature. Coconut oils are great for a variation in taste, and as long as you stick to breakfast "grease" that is made up of healthy fats and natural oils, you can eat as much as you want. Breakfast is a great way to load up on your fats as well because you will predispose your body to burn them off for the rest of the day, a quick twelve-hour metabolism increase that you will only benefit from. If you are the type to wake up with a sweet tooth, the ketogenic reset will not really do that much resetting. All you have to do to make delicious sugary breakfast confections is switch out your sweetener and bready grains. Plenty of keto breakfast snacks are no-bake, which makes them easy to meal prep, and with nut flours instead of wheat flours, you really will not notice a difference. Dark chocolate and small amounts of fruit are some of the tastiest breakfast additions on top of a keto breakfast pancake. To create this tasty and familiar comfort food, all you need is some keto cottage cheese and husk powder. For the oatmeal lovers out there who are wondering where they'll get their fix, it is more than possible to cook up a pot of coconut-based keto oatmeal that goes great with chia seeds and walnuts. Since fruit is limited on the keto diet, smoothies aren't normally your best option for a low-carb breakfast. Integrating vegetables, protein powders, and nuts and seeds into your morning smoothies can make for a delicious keto alternative, without all the added sugar. While you will learn more about "keto coffee" in the section about what to expect when you are eating keto, the second-best way to get a dose of energy first thing in the morning is by eating green vegetables with your eggs. No, not green eggs with your ham – ham is not the best choice for a keto diet. Instead, pair your eggs with spinach, asparagus, green peppers, and scallions for a boost of antioxidants and vitamins. You might already know many breakfast recipes that could be keto with just a few simple tweaks, and that's the beauty of the ketogenic reset: you will not have to reset your mindset in order to get your nutrition. Breakfast is also a great time to indulge in a keto fat bomb for a sweet treat that you will have ample time to burn off. Check out the recipes below for more on how to make keto fat bombs, but for now, let's take a look at lunch.

Keto Lunch Ideas

Lunch is the most notoriously tricky meal to make healthy, easy, and filling, while also managing a job that most likely is not close to a fully stocked keto kitchen. Meal preparation is going to be your biggest help when it comes to making larger, more filling keto meals that have to be higher in volume in order to keep you satisfied. But before you can learn to prepare your lunches in advance, you should probably learn what meals you will be eating. Ketos lunches are often large salads packed with leafy greens and crunchy nuts or Italian-influenced vegetable replacement pasta. If you didn't think you could enjoy a meal of acorn squash ravioli more than beef and cheese, you might be surprised at how hearty, and delicious keto pasta can be. When it comes to lunchtime, you want to aim for recipes that can be made in large batches and served in smaller portions that are reheat-able. Plenty of keto dieters use large casserole dishes like Dutch ovens to cook thickly layered meals that will not leave them hungry by two p.m. Just because bread is off the table doesn't mean that you have to rule out your favorite for lunch though, either. Carbohydrates are easily replaced with Portobello mushrooms, and your BLT doesn't actually need to cut out the B. While turkey bacon is packed with protein and great for breakfast, you are entirely allowed to eat crunchy crispy pork bacon on a keto diet. Lunchtime is playtime for the keto diet, and if you've always wanted to try stuffing a pepper, now is a great time to do so! Warm stuffed peppers with cauliflower rice, spinach, and southwestern jalapenos pack up easily in a lunch box, and if you slice a spaghetti squash in half, you can create the most delicious serving bowl you've ever tasted. Although you should be maintaining a ketogenic diet that is higher in fish than it is in lean protein, chicken is a fabulous way to fill up on hearty lunch meal that will not bust your carbohydrate bank. A word of caution when it comes to chicken, however – even small portions of breast meat tend to be packed with protein. One three-ounce portion, a regularly recommended dietary amount, contains twenty-three grams of protein. That will already put your over your protein limit for the day, so you should take care to measure and weigh your portions of chicken as accurately as possible. Especially if you are planning to exercise in combination with the keto diet, chicken is one lunch protein you will definitely want to stock up on. (Bonus tip: remember to use your freezer when you are purchasing ingredients like vegetables and chicken. Oftentimes you will be able to find sales on bulk items that will work perfectly for meal prepping large entrees. Keeping them frozen in your freezer will stop your groceries from going bad and will help you save money.)

Keto Dinner Entrees

Dinner time, like all meal times on the ketogenic diet, is a fun and delicious way to enjoy your meals and lose more weight than you thought possible. Shrimp and salmon are staples in keto dinner cooking, and you will be happy to know that fish tends to cook in half the time of beef. While you will not be seeing any traditional garlic bread in keto cooking, do not forget your creativity just because you aren't allowed to have croissants. You can easily fashion a keto version of garlic that, surprisingly, is made out of much less bread and much, *much* more cheese. That's right – keto garlic bread is almost solid cheese. Getting creative with your calories definitely pays off. Almost any dinner entrée that you can make with fish is already keto, from seared Mahi Mahi to sashimi. And although you cannot pair any of these meals with regular French fries, or even their high carbohydrate cousin, the sweet potato fry – that's not to say that plenty of keto eaters have not cooked delicious butternut squash wedges tastier than a yellow steak fry. Speaking of fries, you can always enjoy a tasty cheeseburger made from a turkey or salmon patty with a substitute lettuce wedge instead of a bun. This little secret has been a gluten-free hack for decades, and you will most likely be able to find this keto-friendly alternative at most burger restaurants. The secret to delicious keto dinners is all in the spice profile, so stock up on curries, turmeric, paprika, nutmeg, cayenne pepper, chili powder, cumin, and coriander. You will see these spices almost everywhere in keto cooking, and for a good reason – Asian and Middle-Eastern spices are famous for their anti-inflammatory benefits *and* spectacular depths of flavor. Do not forget to substitute cauliflower rice for any carbohydrate sides that you might want to pair with your dinner, and keep fresh black pepper available for any last-minute tastings. Parmesan is also great to keep around, and if you delve more into the world of keto cheeses, you will find that there are plenty of delicious options to keep you cheesy and happy during dinner time. In the event that you have not quite gotten enough fat in your diet yet, one of the best-kept secrets about the keto diet is how to integrate healthy fats into delicious sweet treats. Let's take a look at dessert and some high-fat snacks you will love while eating keto.

Keto Desserts and High Fat Snacks

During your ketogenic reset, you might find it hard at first to get enough fat content packed into your diet to reach ketosis. Many beginners who start out on a keto diet will not reach ketosis simply because they aren't consuming enough, which is a great problem to have when you are trying to lose weight. In order to make sure you reach ketosis quickly, and can then maintain it, you should incorporate high-fat desserts and snacks into your daily routine (but should we really say "should" when it is delicious snacks and treats?). Keto so-called "fat bombs" are made with a simple recipe usually consisting of a butter, like full-fat almond butter or Ghee, any variety of nut flour, essential fatty oils like coconut oil, dark chocolate, salt, and keto-friendly low carbohydrate sugar replacements. Fat bombs can be almost any flavor, from thick and creamy peanut butter to delicious white chocolate crunches flavored with orange extract. Plenty of the fruit flavors that you find in baking are taken from extracts in the first place, so you will not often have to worry about increasing your carbohydrate intake accidentally. Most of the time, fat bombs are made from oils and fats that are either creamy or runny at room temperature, so you will want to make sure that you also make room in the freezer or refrigerator for storage in-between snacking. When it comes to crafting delicious sugar-free keto desserts, replacement sugars are your new best friend. We will go over some of the most popular specific types of sugar replacements in the final chapter, but for now, all you need to know is where you will be able to use them. Keto diet desserts lack bready grains, sweet fruits, and heavy sugar contents, but they are still just as tasty and will not come along with the guilt of eating something processed. You can make almost any cheesecake recipe fit with your keto diet, and the blueberries and raspberries that you normally pair with a cheesecake are perfectly alright in moderation when you are eating keto. Any cake that you can make with grain flour, you can make with nut flour, and there are plenty of full-fat milk alternatives if you do not want to include processed ingredients. Most dark chocolate contains only around thirteen grams of carbs per serving, but if you want to cut your keto carbs down even further, cacao powder and cocoa powder are both great substitutions (with only two grams of net carbs per tablespoons!). Chocolate cakes, mousses, and soufflés will definitely go down easier if you know that they will not spike your blood sugar, result in extra stored fat, or cause damage to your health and weight loss. Keto snacks are about as easy as keto desserts, but ten times faster and twice as portable. When you feel hungry in between meals and you do not have a fat bomb around to help you out, a handful of almonds, hazelnuts, or cashews works like a charm. If you want to spice things up a bit, avocados make great last-minute guacamole when combined with a little bit of salt, pepper, and chopped tomatoes. Although you should not be reaching for berries any time soon, a few blueberries are great for your brain, and they won't ruin your chances at successful ketosis. Choosing natural snacks that are whole and healthy by themselves isn't just easy – it's the best way to get all your natural keto portions while making sure you won't accidentally upset your digestion.

What You Are Allowed to Drink on Keto

If you are at all familiar with the dieting world, or with weight loss in general, you are probably painfully aware that alcohol is a high-calorie no-no for almost all fitness routines. Save the Mediterranean diet. It is normally frowned upon to drink such little liquids that have such high calorie and carbohydrate contents. While the Mediterranean diet does allow you to drink one glass of red wine per night, the science behind the healthy antioxidants present in many varietals of red wine doesn't change the sugar content in each glass. Depending on whether your wine tastes sweet or dry, you could be drinking more glucose than your keto diet is prepared to support, and you do not want to sabotage your ketosis before you even get there. Red wines are typically more likely to be sweet, but as long as you pay attention to the labels, nutritional information, and nutrient percentages, you are allowed to drink any dry red or white wine that does not put you over your daily limit of twenty to thirty grams of carbohydrates (which, if you are conservative, a three-gram-of-carbs glass will not). The even better news for drinking on the keto diet is that almost all pure spirits, like vodka, gin, and whiskey, are free of all carbohydrates. While beer lovers are out of luck on the keto diet because of the high amounts of carbohydrates in each pint, there are plenty of ways to restructure your habits so that you can still enjoy a night off with friends without packing on extra pounds. Plus, as more and more individuals become aware of how unhealthy carbohydrates can be, many companies are focusing on producing great tasting, low carb beverages. Keto is one of the most flexible diets when it comes to drinking, but you will want to make sure that in between any alcoholic beverage, you are drinking water and re-hydrating. It is important to maintain your fluid balance on the keto diet, which we will touch on later in the next chapter – but it is also important to enjoy your diets, and a few extra proteins shakes and fewer calories in the days following a night out will reset your ketogenic reset just fine.

Common Keto Myths

Before we continue discussing the various mechanisms and benefits of the ketogenic diet, there are a few common keto myths that might influence your thinking. One of the most potent myths about the ketogenic diet is that the mechanism of metabolism keto taps into is commonly known as the "starvation mechanism". While this is entirely the truth, the keto diet tends to get a negative reputation based on the false assumption that a keto diet is a way to starve your body into weight loss sustainably. Although the process of cellular respiration that the keto diet forces your body to use is the same mechanism that our bodies tap into when we are starving, the ketogenic diet is an entirely scientific and full-calorie eating program that simply aims to satisfy you and fill you up with a different *source* of nutrition, instead of *lesser amounts* of nutrition. One of the next most influential, and incorrect, myths about the ketogenic diet is that you will not be able to maintain it forever, and you will eventually have to return to metabolizing glucose in order to live. While this myth is not entirely incorrect, it does operate on an incorrect knowledge of the body's mechanisms. It is definitely possible to eat on a ketogenic diet for long periods of time, with careful consideration and medical attention to your body. Many keto dieters choose to eat cyclically because a keto lifestyle can be a bit hard to manage in between work and social life. However, if you have the time to commit to a keto diet that you do not think will interfere with your lifestyle, you have all the more potential to eat on keto for an extended period of time successfully. The other facet of this myth is that most people don't *want* to eat a ketogenic diet for their entire lives. Sometimes, adding in carbohydrates for a week of vacation can be great for the body and for the soul, and if you have already reached your weight loss goals, it is almost silly to continue eating a diet designed to help you shed pounds consistently. While ketone bodies aren't the best for our bloodstreams, yes, that does not mean that a ketogenic diet cannot be functionally integrated into a life-long routine. In case you still have a few more lingering questions about the benefits, or nuances, of a ketogenic reset, here are a few of the most popular questions about the ketogenic diet paired with answers that will clear away any doubts that you have about going keto.

Frequently Asked Keto Questions

A ketogenic diet should never be scary or intimidating because it is simple and natural science. However, any big diet that demands such an involved lifestyle makeover can seem like a bit of a menace. Luckily there are many individuals who have tackled the keto diet before you, and just like scientific research, each one has helped us better understand the mechanisms of the keto diet. Until now, you've had to sit back and listen quietly to the details of a lifestyle change that you might not have been entirely sure about making. Now that you understand the significant positive benefits of a ketogenic diet, you probably have more than a few clarifying questions. Let's address some of the most frequently asked questions about the keto diet and dispel any remaining concerns preventing you from going keto and starting the next phase of your fitness.

- Is it normal to feel fatigued on the keto diet?

It is normal to feel fatigued on the ketogenic diet for the first three to seven days, although you should only feel weak for three to five. The keto diet begins by purging your body of harmful carbohydrates and sugars that have built up in your bloodstream. Just like any mildly addictive substance, sugar causes a bit of a hangover, and you start off the keto diet with a fatigued weakness that's a result of your body craving sugar. Do not worry, though – you will not be in sugar withdrawal for long. Drink plenty of water, eat enough healthy fats to keep yourself satisfied, and try to get enough sleep and you should feel better soon. Once your body adjusts to metabolizing fats instead of metabolizing carbohydrates, you will re-adjust to normal function. If your fatigue continues for longer than seven days, immediately consult a doctor and slowly begin to eat your normal diet.

· How long does the keto diet take to work?

The keto diet, like any diet, works differently from person to person, but on average, a body that has been properly cleansed of carbohydrates and sugars in preparation for keto can reach ketosis in two days. While we will talk more in-depth about reaching ketosis in Chapter Four, for now, you should keep in mind that all your diet goals should be realistic. It is only healthy for an adult person to lose between one and two pounds per week, and if you are determining whether or not keto is "working" for you by how many pounds you have lost - make sure you aren't taxing your body with unhealthy eating conditions. Ketogenic diets cannot usually be sustained without periodic breaks to help relax your system, and so most individuals operate on a three to four-week ketogenic cycle in between more loosely structured eating days. This cycle of on-and-off ketogenic eating can continue for as long as you healthily and safely pay attention to your body's needs.

- How much weight will I lose on the keto diet?

On any diet, it is only safe to lose between one and two pounds per day without placing undue stress on your heart muscles. Counting your calories is the best way to make sure you are losing weight, but the ketogenic diet will naturally help you shed pounds even if you do not eat on a calorie deficit. As a lifestyle, keto dieters tend always to be smaller than individuals who eat more carbs, and so your weight loss on keto is really very dependent on your own course of action.

- What foods do you eat on a keto diet?

On a ketogenic diet, you will be eating foods that

are low in carbohydrates and high in healthy fats. While that might seem self-explanatory, the ketogenic diet goes deeper than just omitting grains, processed foods, and starchy legumes. Plenty of healthy vegetables and fruits are packed with carbohydrates, and while this is not necessarily bad for you, on a ketogenic diet, you want to make sure that you are limiting your sugar intake no matter whether that sugar is healthy or not. Fruits that are larger than your palm, orange, or yellow tend to be filled with natural sugars that will trigger your body to revert to catabolizing glucose instead of catabolizing fat. Vegetables that are high in starch and fiber-like sweet potatoes, black beans, and chickpeas are also high in carbohydrates, so you will want to stick to leafy greens instead.

· Will the keto diet help me lose belly fat?

Yes, in fact, the ketogenic diet is scientifically proven to be one of the best diets for targeting stubborn belly fat, love handles, and limbic fat around your internal organs. The keto diet rewires your energy-harvesting mechanisms to digest fat instead of sugar, but our bodies love sugar far too much. During the first few weeks of the keto diet, your body will search all over your body for fat stores of leftover glucose to catabolize. Tough stored fat deep down in your fat cells tends to clump in hard-to-work-out places, like your lower abdominals. Dieting is virtually the only way to convince your body to dip into these well-stored fat reserves, and the keto diet specifically is designed to target just the exact stubborn fat that you are looking to lose.

· Should I consider tomatoes a fruit or vegetable while eating keto?

Ketogenic diets can be tricky if you aren't sure whether or not you are allowed to eat something – but simply now knowing the answer should never stop you from trying new things! The keto diet considers a tomato to be a vegetable, in the sense that the carbohydrate content of one serving of tomatoes is much closer to the carbohydrate content of the same size serving of broccoli. The carb content of the same serving size of bananas would be far too high, and so you are allowed to eat tomatoes like you would eat a vegetable on keto, instead of like you would eat fruits. (Consider also: even though ears of corn look, and feel, and seem, like vegetables – they are actually grains, and they are packed with carbohydrate sugars that will sabotage your journey to ketosis.)

· What is the difference between carbs and fiber?

Fiber is a type of carbohydrate normally found in high concentrations in fruits, vegetables, and legumes like beans and nuts. Although our bodies cannot technically digest fiber, it is an important component of our diets nonetheless. Fiber helps to slow down your digestion and clear out blockages that build up in your small and large intestines. Because we cannot digest fiber, it picks up and cleans out the toxins left behind in our digestive tract as it moves and then removes them as waste. This is one of the reasons that you will learn to subtract the amount of dietary fiber present on a nutritional label from the amount of total carbohydrates. Since you cannot digest fiber, the grams of "dietary" fiber in the food that you eat will never count toward your daily carb total. The leftover grams of carbohydrates after this subtraction problem are your net carbs, the only carbohydrates that your body will digest and absorb into your bloodstream.

· Is a ketogenic diet vegan?

One of the most attractive things about the ketogenic reset diet is that you can either choose to eat vegan, vegetarian, or pescetarian as well as fully carnivorous and reap similar results. Plenty of ketogenic eaters decide to go along with a vegan keto diet simply because of the unhealthy processing methods and hormonal additives that are found in animal products. But you certainly are not required to eat vegan, although there are many delicious nutrients found in foods like eggs and fish that you might have to supplement if you do not choose to eat them. Keto is always flexible, and it is incredibly easy to spot animal products even in regular keto recipes that you can switch out.

· Will I lose muscle on the keto diet?

The short answer to whether or not you will lose muscle on the keto diet is yes. While most of us are not quite at the point where this muscle loss would be significant, if you are beginning with a stronger and more built frame, you will likely see decreases in your muscle mass almost immediately. A ketogenic diet simply doesn't support massive gains and large, carbohydrate-thirsty muscles. There are many ways, however, that the keto diet can be altered in order to work with higher intensity physical activity, and if you want to keep your muscle mass (or continue to build upon it), you can easily carbohydrate-load before a workout which we will learn about in the last chapter.

· Does a keto diet cause kidney stones?

Diets that are higher in protein than we are used to are always more likely to give our bodies kidney stones, but as long as you are maintaining your potassium levels, you should not develop kidney stones on the keto diet. When the keto diet was first created in the early nineteen twenties, some early participants showed signs of kidney stones, but modern science is easily able to manage the possible causes associated with a high-fat diet.

· Why do you need to take salt on the keto diet?

Speaking of kidney stones, one of the reasons that early implications of the keto diet tended to cause kidney stones in younger patients is because they lacked enough electrolytes. Sodium, potassium, calcium, and magnesium are some of the most important electrolytes for your body, and if you are drinking lots of water, these water-soluble molecules will do just that: dissolve in water. If you are not getting enough sodium from the foods that you are eating, you should carefully supplement your ketogenic reset with sodium to make sure that your body is able to balance your water levels chemically. If you want to learn more about why water is so important to your keto diet, skip down to Chapter Four.

·   Is counting calories part of the keto diet?

Technically, counting calories is not a required part of the ketogenic diet. However, if you will remember, any sort of weight loss is really scientifically determined by a calorie deficit, and if you are not operating on a deficit, it is likely that you will not lose as much weight as you possibly could. When you are eating a ketogenic diet, it is best to eat on a calorie deficit of no more than thirty-five hundred calories per week or the equivalent of one pound of fat. On average, healthy human adult can lose between one and two pounds per week at a healthy rate. If you want to maximize your weight loss on a keto diet, counting your calories is a great way to do so.

· Can I afford the keto diet?

Unlike diets like the Mediterranean diet that tend to demand expensive ingredients that can be hard to find in your local grocery stores, the keto diet is very easily accessible for all tax brackets. Many grocery stores will already sell the natural ingredients you will be looking for, and when it comes to buying produce and non-processed, unpackaged ingredients in bulk, you will probably find that your receipt each week gets cheaper and cheaper. Keto dieters are sometimes known to spend even less than the modern adult who eats out and grocery shops only occasionally. The value of a dollar definitely goes further on keto.

· Are there different types of keto diet?

The keto diet itself is not just another low-carbohydrate regime, although there *are* plenty of those – from the Atkin's diet to paleo and Whole30. What sets the keto diet apart from other low-carb diets is its emphasis on living a sustainable, and long-term, weight loss lifestyle. This means that yes, that are plenty of different types of the keto diet, but each one focuses on changing your diet and exercise routines to fit your lifestyle. The most common version of the ketogenic diet is a breakdown of five to ten percent carbs, fifteen to twenty percent proteins, and a standard seventy-five percent fat content. However, you can choose to take on a low-impact keto diet that will simply help you shed pounds, water weight, and processed sugars that doesn't require full-time keto. This low-impact version of the diet operates in a cycle of keto days and classic "cheat" days when you are allowed to consume fats, proteins, and carbs in a 25/25/50 ratio. For athletes, a keto diet higher in carbohydrates on a regular basis is probably the best course of action, and this tends to look like a sixty-five to seventy percent fat intake paired with a ten to fifteen percent carbohydrate intake.

What Keto Will Do For You

The Medical Benefits of Keto

Type 2 Diabetes

As we touched on in the introductory section of this guide, the Atkin's diet and keto diet, in turn, were developed to control a certain autoimmune disease that science has yet to find a cure for. Parkinson's disease, Alzheimer's, and certain cases of epilepsy are debilitating to those they afflict, and it is a revolutionary notion that what you eat can help better fuel your body to target a problem. When it comes to the ketogenic diet, the greatest health benefits are associated with eating a low carbohydrate diet in general. Choosing to cut out excess glucose from your diet will immediately allow your blood sugar to self-regulate, which is an attractive benefit for anyone suffering from Type 2 diabetes. Type 2 diabetes, unlike Type 1 diabetes, is normally contracted later in life because of risk factors like high cholesterol and atherosclerosis caused by high blood sugar. When you eat too much-saturated fat or glucose, your body cannot produce enough insulin to regulate the level of sugar in your blood. Insulin is produced by your pancreas in order to help your cells obtain sugar. Sugar is broken down in the cytoplasm of your cells, but glucose is a large molecule, and your cell walls are closely knit in order to contain their organelles. Each cell has to make sure structures like your mitochondria and ribosomes are safely contained, so insulin helps your cells safely open while they do so in order to facilitate passage of glucose molecules. Your pancreas stimulates insulin release when your blood sugar levels rise, commonly after you eat. Individuals with Type 2 diabetes struggle to produce enough insulin, and so their cells are unable to open and receive glucose molecules. Your blood sugar is almost always high when you have Type 2 diabetes, and you should be able to see why a diet that is low in glucose would be beneficial to this disorder. If your diet functions to regulate how much sugar you eat, your body will not have to regulate how much sugar is present in your bloodstream. Unfortunately, Type 2 diabetes often can only be treated with oral or intravenous insulin infusions, which will only become more and more necessary as the disease progresses untreated. Regulating how much sugar is in your bloodstream naturally will help your body rely less and less on external insulin, and the healing effects of an anti-inflammatory keto diet will help abate some of the symptoms of Type 2 diabetes.

Inflammation, Depression, and Anxiety

"Anti-inflammatory" is a phrase which means anything that promotes the relaxation of swollen or inflamed vessels, and it is one of the many other benefits of a keto diet for dieters who have something other than Type 2 diabetes. Anti-inflammatory food groups are also, coincidentally, food groups that are high in whole natural fats and fatty acids. Inflammation occurs with more than Type 2 diabetes – in fact, inflammation comes with everything from arthritis, which is obvious, to depression, in which inflammation can occur internally and unnoticed. Natural oils, small berries, nuts, and the keto diet staple, green vegetables, can all help calm inflammation throughout your body. Eating a keto diet can also help manage the symptoms of many mental disorders, which is a lesser studied phenomenon but very tangible nonetheless. Mood disorders like anxiety and depression, as well as more serious afflictions like bipolar disorder and schizophrenia, can all be caused *and aggravated by* inflammation. Stress and anxious feelings ramp up our sympathetic nervous system, the half of our nervous system that controls our fight-or-flight response. While it is not entirely known why stress and fight-or-flight hormones cause intense inflammation, many suffer from general anxiety, bipolar disorder, and chronic depression have shown improvements on a keto diet. Part of this improvement could be linked to the ketogenic reset's ability to refresh your metabolism. When your body is able to function efficiently and effectively, it is more likely that you are going to be able to circulate all the proper nutrients and energy to all the proper places. A well-fed brain that is low on stress can better cope with negative emotions and anxious situations. A ketogenic diet does not just function to abate the symptoms of diseases you already have, however. Eating in a keto style can be preventive in fighting many different types of cancers as well — because it physically starves them. Cancer cells need glucose to grow, and if there is not any present, they die. Mutated cancer cells are unable to catabolize ketone bodies as our cells can. But that's not all. Because a keto diet tends to be free of highly processed fats and oils, unhealthy chemical additives, and harmful hormones used in packaging, you are less likely to be exposed to the carcinogens in processed foods. Carcinogens are anything that can cause cancer, and it is not just a cynical phrase to think that they are present in almost everything. From sugary soda drinks to "all-natural" juices and ketchup, many preserved and sealed foods are packed with unhealthy disaccharide sugars. Chemical additives will always contribute to the likelihood that you will develop certain mutating cells, but if you eat a daily diet that doesn't include additives in the first place, you are much less likely to develop uncontrollable cells later on.

Fatty Liver Disease

Fatty liver disease is about what the name suggests it is – your liver stores fat, and when you store too much, you created the condition of a fatty liver. Most of the time, a fatty liver is diagnosed as a result of external sources, like drinking too much alcohol, eating too many saturated fats, and clogging your bloodstream with sugar. Fatty livers are typically any liver with ten percent or more fat content, but you will likely have been diagnosed by your doctor before you yourself realize you have it. Fatty livers are easily controlled, and actually, can be reversed – by eating a diet high in healthy fats. Although it is a bit of a strange and unjustified solution, fatty livers are a strange and unknown phenomenon that scientists have had to study based on what diseases a fatty liver acts most like. Coincidentally, a fatty liver is connected to high blood pressure, high cholesterol, increased sodium in the bloodstream, Type 1 diabetes, and general obesity. All of these things can be regulated, and fixed, by a ketogenic diet; although scientists do not know why a ketogenic diet also regulates and fixes a fatty liver. The predominant theory is that a fatty liver is more intimately connected to obesity and the effects on an unhealthy diet in the same way that your more delicate internal organs also are – your heart, arteries, and pancreas and just as susceptible to the dangers of high-carb, high saturated fat diets. As long as you are regulating your diet appropriately, and combining your ketogenic reset with daily mild exercise totaling at least thirty minutes with an elevated heart rate, you should see the same weight loss effects on your liver that you do on your body. A fatty liver does not have to become a life-threatening health issue, and as long as you are taking the proper precautions to prevent it, you should be well able to maintain a healthy liver on a keto diet *before* you have to reverse the damage.

Pre-Keto Health Precautions

Like any diet or medical decision that will affect

your entire body, starting a keto diet is not always the best course of action for those of us with certain health concerns. Especially when it comes to the restrictive and sometimes rigorous dieting routine of the keto lifestyle, it is important for you to understand and listen to your body. Any diet that operates on the basis of restricting what you can and cannot eat has the potential to trigger past eating disorders in individuals with a history or to trigger the development of eating disorders in individuals who have not shown symptoms in the past. The key thing to keep in mind when it comes to the keto diet is that science is science, and science also says that your body will not be healthy if you do not work to consume essential nutrients actively. The keto diet is a weight loss lifestyle, designed to teach you how to eat for the rest of your life healthily. If you are considering a keto diet in order to drop pounds for any reason other than the health of your body, mind, and lifestyle, it simply will not be a healthy regime for you to take on. The keto diet can also be unhealthy for individuals with certain pre-existing medical conditions. For example, while a keto diet has been proven to help with Type 2 diabetes, individuals suffering from a lifetime of Type 1 diabetes should absolutely avoid eating a keto diet.

How to Be Successful at Keto

Content Warning: The following chapter, while informative and helpful for those seeking knowledgeable dieting advice, could be triggering for individuals who are struggling or have struggled with disordered eating. If you are uncomfortable or anxious discussing targeted caloric weight loss, nutritional numbers, or weight goals and loss tips, skip down to Chapter Five.

Counting Your Calories

Losing weight might seem like a difficult and often unsolvable puzzle, but it really boils down to a simple science: if you eat fewer calories than your body needs to burn, you will lose weight. Many people integrate this idea into their fitness and diet regimes in order to make sure that they end each week with a calorie deficit. Calories deficits are, realistically, the most scientific way to make sure you are losing weight. But simply eating less doesn't always do the trick, just like working out all the time without a healthy diet will not change your weight. In order to make sure your keto diet is working effectively to help you lose weight, you are going to want to count your calories in combination with a fitness regime (although we will touch more on exercise in Chapter Six). The science behind counting calories is the same for every diet, no matter what types of foods you are eating. Losing weight, remember, is as simple as eating fewer calories per day then you need to sustain daily activity. If you chose to create a calorie deficit with a workout, that is just as effective, but if you want to be sure at the start that you are eating for weight loss, you should count your physical calories. One pound of fat tends to equal around thirty-five hundred calories, which means that after burning that amount, you will have lost one pound.

Anyone trying to lose weight should aim to create a thirty-five hundred calorie deficit in their diet each week, with a goal of losing between one and two pounds per week. With rough estimates like these, it is important to keep in mind that weight loss is also highly dependent upon age, height, sex, weight, and health history. You might not lose as much as two pounds in the first few weeks of your deficit, or you might lose more than you would have expected. Depending on your old eating and drinking habits, you could lose more or less. The best way to track your weight loss and make sure you are losing weight at a healthy rate is to consult with your doctor. However, weighing yourself with a bathroom scale at home can be just as helpful. If you are not the type of person who weighs themselves every morning, do not worry – it is effective enough to weigh yourself once at the beginning, and once at the end, of each week. Scales do not have to be intimidating, but if you aren't their biggest fan, make sure to stay tuned for Chapter Seven – your scale could be your new favorite thing. In the meantime, let's talk about why keeping track of how much *of what* you eat is just as important as keeping track of how much you eat.

"Macros", "Micros", and Eating for Ketosis

Counting your calories is all well and good, but think about diets that are high in processed foods and unhealthy fats; you can cap those calories at a perfect thirty-five hundred deficit, but will you lose weight if the calories you are consuming are empty? The answer, of course, is no. A calorie deficit simply will not work if you are not ensuring that you are first and foremost getting the proper nutrition from a healthy source. That's where "macros" and "micros" come in. These two abbreviations stand for our macronutrients and our micronutrients, the essential chemicals that our body's need to function. Each macronutrient and micronutrient is necessary for our daily function, and it is sometimes shocking how few people are deficient in more than a few areas of their diet. When it comes to eating a keto diet, it is not just important that you count your macros and micros; you should also be keeping track of your daily net carbs, for every meal, snack, and drink you consume. Keto is a very scientific process, and if either of these measurements are off, you will not be able to reach let alone maintain your ketosis-fueled weight loss. Here are the best ways to keep count of your macro and micronutrients, and the best ways to make sure that your net carbs aren't sabotaging your hard work.

Macronutrients

"Macros" and "micros" might sound like intimidating body-builder slang you never thought that you would use, but macronutrients are much simpler to understand than their name suggests. There are only three macronutrients, and they happen to be the three types of fuel that we have been discussing already. Carbohydrates, proteins, and fats (or, scientifically, "lipids"), are the three macronutrients that your body needs to function. The actual word micronutrient means something along the lines of "necessary for life" – and they are. We need carbohydrates, proteins, and fats to survive, but we do not need them all in the same amounts. You know that eating too many carbohydrates can result in storing too much extra glycogen, and even eating too much fat creates the ketone body bi-product of a low-carb diet. Both of these extremes aren't where our body likes to exist, but keto is much healthier than obesity. When it comes to tracking your macronutrients for a keto diet, there are a few industry professionals that have luckily gone before you to help decide on proportions. The classical ketogenic diet only allows five percent of your diet to come from carbohydrates, while seventy-five percent goes towards healthy fats, and only twenty percent should consist of protein. Think back to when we discussed how a keto diet has to have oxygen in order to complete cellular respiration with fatty acids instead of glucose; if you are only consuming five percent of carbohydrates per day, you aren't going to be able to do a lot of muscle-building exercises. Athletes are a great example of how the keto diet's macronutrients do not have to be so strict all the time: if you need more carbohydrates, you can calculate your macros intake based on your biological statistics (age, height, sex, etc.) and your level of physical activity. Chapter Six will teach you the exact numbers for healthily carbo-loading your keto diet, but for now, you should make sure that your keto proportions do not exceed thirty grams of net carbohydrates per day, and that your protein intake never sinks below fifteen percent. Protein works to help you maintain muscle growth and regeneration, and gives your body the fuel it needs to build new protein. But your main focus when it comes to your macronutrients is to make sure you are eating as little carbohydrates as possible while getting as many healthy fats from natural sources as possible with protein filling in the gaps. Tracking your macronutrients is much easier with a food scale and during meal prep, but you will learn all those skills in due time. For now, keep those portions in mind as we move into discussing how to track your net carbohydrates for maximum keto success.

Counting Your Net Carbs

When you are eating on a keto diet, you want to make sure that you are consuming as little daily carbohydrates as possible in order to reach ketosis. Ketosis, remember, is the state of burning fat instead of burning sugar for energy. Once you have reached ketosis, your body will seek out its own stored sugar supply in order to burn off all the rest of your carbohydrates. This is one of the key reasons that the keto diet is so effective at facilitating weight loss. Every human body has a certain amount of stored sugar in the form of glycogen that is present in our liver cells, muscle cells, and fat cells. We store glucose in the form of the molecule glycogen in order to keep it safe and packaged like perishable foods for use later on. As your body starts to run out of a consistent supply of glucose, it will start to seek out your stored supply of glycogen. If you have ever tried to get rid of what is commonly called "stubborn fat", you might be familiar with your stored supplies of glycogen. Stored supplies of glycogen in fat cells are difficult to get at on the surface, and if your body has an ample supply of glucose to burn on the hand, this becomes the fat that is the most difficult to target during weightlifting exercises. If your diet has no glucose, even without a workout, your metabolism will seek out the glucose it likes to burn the most that has been locked away in your fat cells. Lower abdominal fat, fat around the midsection, and stubborn limbic fat that clumps around your internal organs are all hard to reach places that cardio and weights cannot burn. In order to make sure that you are reaping the benefits of a fat-burning diet, you have to limit the amount of glucose you eat per day, so you will not trigger your glucose-burning mechanisms. Keto diets tend to operate in a range of thirty or fewer grams of carbohydrates per day, with most individuals seeking to eat closer to twenty grams. You never want to eat over thirty-five grams of total carbs, but you will notice on some nutritional labels, plenty of foods are packed with tens of hundreds of carbohydrates. Nutritional labels are never easy to read, but especially when it comes to carbohydrates, there are certain sugars that our body is physically unable to digest. These carbs run right through our systems and do not add any digested sugars to our bloodstream. When you read a nutritional label, you want to make sure you know how to calculate how many of these usable carbs or net carbs, our body actually manages to absorb. The equation for finding net carbohydrates is simple, but not readily obvious: in order to calculate net carbs, subtract the amount of dietary fibers on the nutritional label from the amount of total carbohydrates. This number will give you your net carbs, and it is almost always a smaller number than the one that the label tells you. These net carbs will directly affect your body's ability to reach ketosis, and so you want to make sure that you aren't eating more than twenty grams per day of net carbs. Luckily, many ketogenic recipes and fitness regimes are designed to reflect your limited carb intake, so you will be able to find nutritional information and calculated net carbs for plenty of keto lifestyle tips. Now that you know how to keep track of your macronutrients and your net carbohydrates, there is one more important source of nutrients that you need to cover on a keto diet.

Micronutrients

Their name might already indicate that these nutrients are going to be a bit more detailed than your macronutrients, but do not worry – micronutrients aren't complicated at all, but they are definitely worth your time. Remember how your body is unable to function without a certain amount of each macronutrient? Micronutrients work much the same, but there are seven of them that are widely recommended and over twenty-nine in total. Yes, twenty-nine. But you know the micronutrients in much more familiar terms than you might think. Like "macronutrients", "micronutrients" is just a very scientific word for your vitamins and minerals. From B, C, and vitamin D3 to zinc and calcium, vitamins and minerals are essential to a healthy functioning body. The seven micronutrients that you need as recommended by most government medical agencies and doctors are vitamin B12, vitamin D3, vitamin A, iron, zinc, iodine, and calcium. While most of these vitamins and minerals can be found in a general multivitamin, it is a smart idea while you are eating a keto diet to supplement each micronutrient individually. To this list, you should also add omega-3 fatty acids, vitamin k, magnesium, and potassium supplements alongside sodium tablets (a relationship we will discuss a little later on in Chapter Eight). Your keto diet might at times cause your cholesterol levels to spike if you aren't careful about the amount of natural, whole fats that you are eating. Too many saturated, unhealthy fats will cause a build-up of plaque in the arteries around your heart as a result of too much bad cholesterol.

Beginning Keto the Right Way

Preparing your body for an intense keto cleanse and lifestyle makeover is not as involved as you might think, but it is definitely as important. Priming your body to catabolize fats instead of carbohydrates is going to be a long process if you are used to eating a diet full of grains and sugars. The best way to prepare your body for a ketogenic reset is to slowly start weaning yourself off of carbohydrates, processed sugars, unhealthy fruits, and too much protein. Think about the last time you ordered out at a restaurant. Your entrée likely came with sides, and you likely did not pick the leafy green option. Beginning to integrate a keto diet into your lifestyle is as easy as making small, healthier choices that will lessen the impact of an entirely new diet, and switching out your carbs is a great way to start. Next, you will want to take a look at your drinking habits. Many of us consume more sugar than we realize in our beverages, and if you are not careful, this is one of the things that can intensify the symptoms of your carbohydrate flu. Coffee drinkers who put sugar in their morning cups will definitely want to take a look at the recipe for keto-friendly bulletproof coffee a few weeks before transitioning into a full keto diet. If you do not want to add oil to your brew just yet, try substituting a natural, artificial sweetener like Stevia instead. If your fridge is packed to the brim with sugary Coca Cola, you might want to try keto coffee sooner rather than later – you can make an iced version that is just as delicious if you prepare it the night before in a warm saucepan and keep it refrigerated overnight. People who get their energy from sugar get hit the hardest when you are forced to cut out soda and juice on a keto diet. Slowly allowing your body to get used to drinking water with squeezed citrus like lemon or orange will help prevent crabbiness, migraines, fatigue, and cravings during your first week of keto. Another helpful tip for jumping into keto fully prepared is to try and regulate your sleeping patterns. The ketogenic diet is famous for its ability to help you sleep like a rock once you have reached ketosis, but during the carbohydrate flu stage, you might find yourself hit with a bought of keto insomnia. Dieters who reach ketosis tend to report that they naturally wake up earlier, and fall asleep earlier than they did before they began the keto diet. If you stay up late, and sleep in late, you might want to consider resetting your sleeping habits before you start eating low-carb; otherwise, you might have to endure a few more sleepless nights before your body settles into catabolizing only fats. The biggest catch about the keto diet, and the uncomfortable symptoms of the keto-carb flu is that the human body can really only maintain its stores of sugar for two days. Although a regular carbohydrate flu tends to last between three and five days, some dieters have reported whole weeks of symptoms related to carb withdrawal. Scientifically, if you take the time to slowly prepare your body for at least two to three weeks before engaging in a full-blown keto diet, you will be able to reach ketosis faster, and start losing weight faster, than individuals who have not prepared. There's a reason why most individuals on a keto diet take the time to study the details and understand the mechanisms, and that reason is that it works. Taking the time to ensure that your body is primed and ready to take on the keto diet will allow keto to work its magic, and you will wonder why you hadn't started eating low-carb sooner.

Are You in Ketosis?

Speaking of only two days, you might be wondering why this whole "fat-burning mechanism" called ketosis is so effective, and so seemingly easy to achieve if so many dieters aren't able to get there.

Ketosis is easy to achieve, yes, but as with everything that has to do with the human body, your own personal statistics have a huge impact on your body's ability to reach and maintain ketosis. If you are entering into a keto diet with more stored body fat than someone else, it is definitely going to take you longer to enter into a state of ketosis. Your body's first course of action after you have purged your water weight and stopped supplying it with glucose is to search out whatever sugar you have stored on your person. Your body will use up the stored supplies of glycogen in your muscles and your liver before moving on to catabolize the glycogen in your fat cells. These areas, remember, are often your tougher to target sections - your front lower abdominals, your lower back love handles, and the limbic fat around your vital internal organs. One of the best ways to determine if your body is close to ketosis is by monitoring your weight and your weight loss regions. If you start to notice that you are losing weight without putting in more effort at the gym, or if you start to notice that areas of more stubborn fat are shrinking, it is likely that you are close to ketosis. However, for those of us who are more scientific, there are few more obvious indicators of a full-blown state of ketosis. Although stinky breath is a less attractive side effect of ketosis that we will tackle in the next chapter, you should also experience a lovely wave of mental clarity along with maximizing your fat breakdown. As your brain begins to rely on ketone bodies for energy, instead of running on glucose fumes, you should feel the mental fog of your carbohydrate flu begin to dissipate. On the subject of ketone bodies, if you want to be incredibly exact about whether or not your body has reached ketosis, there are plenty of home test kits that can measure the ketone levels in your blood. For those of us who are not squeamish, blood testing with an electronic device is a reliable and concrete way to determine if you are in ketosis. Word of warning, however – be careful that you measure for more than just one of the three types of molecules present in a ketone body; oftentimes electronic blood meters are designed for diabetes patients, and will only tell you one of your three levels of ketones. If you are a bit squeamish around blood, you can always use a urine test strip to monitor your ketone levels that way. Each strip is fairly self-explanatory, and although they aren't as accurate as a blood test, a urine strip will still give you a definitive answer. The third and final way for you to test the ketone levels in your blood is with a breathalyzer device. Ketones are present in high quantities in your breath when you reach ketosis, causing the famous "keto mouth" that most dieters combat with chewing gum and mints. A breathalyzer device works similarly to a blood tester, and you should be able to easily track your ketone readings in times between meals, drinking, and brushing your teeth.

What to Expect When You are Eating Keto

The Carbohydrate Flu Explained

The keto diet is not just a three-week eating plan that aims to help you cut down before a big event. Eating for a ketogenic reset means that you are digging down to the stubborn toxins your body can't purge in order to start fresh – and that is not necessarily the most fun process. Most of us are used to eating sugars, whether processed or unprocessed, in incredible amounts each day that we often are not aware of. Sugars (particularly processed sugars) are hidden everywhere both in places you would expect them to be and places you would be shocked to find such high a content. Some of the most shocking culprits of added sugar are inconsequential foods like salad dressings, barbecue sauces, and low fat products that ramp up their sugar content to account for their terrible low fat taste. Because we are so used to consuming mass amounts of sugar, our bodies tend to experience a kind of sugar withdrawal when we first begin to purge our system of glucose. Sugar is a highly addictive substance, but scientists are not entirely sure why. It is obvious that the cultural presence of sugar in our diets since birth has some effect on our constant need for the substance into adulthood, but the fact remains that even if we do not know why we crave sugar, we crave it. The first week or so of the keto diet might have you feeling tired, cranky, nauseous, sweaty or too cold, and unable to regulate your digestion. This is sometimes jokingly referred to as "the keto flu", but it is a phenomenon experienced in plenty of other low carbohydrate diets. Our bodies become desperate for sugar during their initial carbohydrate drought, and you could even experience such withdrawal symptoms as headaches, difficulty sleeping, and joint and muscle aches. The initial severity of your keto, or carb, flu will depend on how much of your diet consisted of carbohydrates before you began the diet. If you are a person who regularly depends on sodas, pastries, and processed or added sugars, your keto flu will most likely be worse than someone who began the diet eating mostly fruits and veggies, with the occasional whole grains. One of the best ways to combat this keto flu is to try and slowly eliminate, or cut back on, your sugar intake before you begin the keto diet. Although this is not a necessary step to make sure your keto diet is effective, even if you are used to two sugars in your coffee in the morning you will get a headache during the first week. The carbohydrate flu, however, is just a mild form of addictive withdrawal, and you will be happy to know that the symptoms tend to abate in three to five days, lasting no longer than a week for most individuals who keep themselves hydrated and implicate a few counteractive health measures (which we will teach you in the next two sections). Stay strong and keep your diet carbohydrate-free for the first few days, and your ketogenic reset will be more or less smooth sailing.

Taking Care of Your Internal Organs

Any time you are training your body to run a process that adds acid to your blood is most likely going to have some side effects for your internal organs. Keto diets are also vastly different in proportion from what most of us are used to, which means you will be experiencing some form of digestive distress, for probably a few different reasons. However, like everything that the keto diet promotes, there are plenty of scientific ways to biologically help your organs weather the storm that is a keto diet. First and foremost, one of the most common intestinal issues associated with the keto diet is diarrhea. When you are eating a diet that is very high in fatty foods, your stomach needs extra enzymes to help digest a large amount of fat you aren't used to. These digestive enzymes that breakdown fat are called "bile", and bile is produced by the liver but stored in your gallbladder. You can imagine that by the middle of a three-week ketogenic diet, your gallbladder is one of the most over-taxed organs in your body, because you are producing, storing, and then flushing out massive amounts of bile. While this does negatively affect your bowels by making them runny and loose, you might be at a lower risk of developing gallstones. The keto diet tends to put your gallbladder to work, and if you can manage the symptoms of your runny bowels with water, fiber, and protein, you can absolutely eat a keto diet that helps flush out your gallbladder without too many bathroom trips. If you have already had gallstones in your life, eating a diet high in fat could have both a positive and negative effect, so you should consult with your doctor before transitioning out of eating carbohydrates. An easy way to help your body combat gallstones is by drinking lemon water. Yes, lemon water. First thing in the morning, lemon juice acts as a revitalizer for your digestive system after a night of sleep – but it is not just healthy to drink in the morning. On a keto diet, in order to help your body breakdown and flush out gallstones, you should drink at least five glasses of lemon water per day. If you want to really clean out your gallbladder in order to maintain a more effective (and comfortable) ketosis, you can also perform what is called a "gallbladder cleanse". Although the scientific verdict is still out on whether or not flushing your body with fruit juices, water, and laxative olive oil actually helps break up gall stones – there are definitely more than a few confirmed cases.

How to Detox Your Liver and Gallbladder

As always, you should consult with your doctor before beginning a cleanse or detox that is designed to target your internal environment. It is worth it to note. However, that of all the cleanses and detoxes that you can perform at home, a liver and gallbladder cleanse uses the highest concentration of natural ingredients that will not have a damaging effect on your body. Especially for women eating on the keto diet, a liver and gallbladder cleanse will help prevent the gall stones that you are more likely to contract. The most common way to perform a gallbladder and liver cleanse is by sectioning off one to two days per week in which you can freely eat and drink. Luckily you will already have eliminated processed sugars, carbohydrates, saturated and trans fats, and processed grains and oils from your diet, so the first step of a normal gall bladder cleanse doesn't apply to you. Eating a diet high in fats will naturally promote the health of your gall bladder by consistently demanding it to be flushed out and refilled with bile. Once these food groups are entirely removed from your diet, you can slowly begin to detox your gall bladder and liver by either one of two methods. The first, and more enjoyable, style of gallbladder cleanses instructs you to eat one green apple with breakfast and one green apple with lunch, while drinking alternating glasses of vegetable juice and apple juice throughout the day. At five p.m., this style of gall bladder and liver detox will not make you take straights shot of olive oil, but you do still have to consume it before bed. For this cleanse, you will want to drink a cocktail consisting of nine milliliters of lemon juice and eighteen milliliters of olive oil every fifteen minutes until you have drunk approximately eight ounces of olive oil. If you'd prefer to go about your day and then take care of your olive oil shots all at once, you can also choose to detox your internal organs by fasting for twelve hours, and then at five p.m., drinking a ratio of one to four tablespoons of lemon juice to olive oil. Again, you will have to repeat this step every fifteen minutes until you have swallowed at least eight ounces of olive oil. Keep in mind that gallbladder and liver cleanses like this aren't necessarily proven science, but olive oil is a natural digestive stimulant, and you will definitely notice the cleansing powers of consuming so much is this short style. Both the olive oil and the acidic chemicals found in apples help to calm inflammation in your system, which also likely has soothing effects on an irritated gall bladder. If you do not want to engage in an entire liver and gall bladder cleanse, there are plenty of ways that you can promote the health of these organs without a detox. Bone broth is one of the best ways to detoxify your liver, as are garlic cloves, broccoli, and beets. Naturally, detoxifying foods combined with lemon juice will also soothe more of your body than just your liver and gall bladder. Plus, there is no better time to drink healthy apple juice or consume more healthy fats than on a ketogenic diet. And if your internal organs feel better, as a result, you will only be happier while you eat a ketogenic diet.

"Keto Mouth" and Fruity Acid Breath

It is no surprise that there are a few negative side effects to switching your body's natural biological mechanisms, but one of the strangest symptoms of a diet low in carbohydrates is bad breath. Although keto dieters do not necessarily refer to it as *bad* breath, there is a certain "fruity" and unpleasant scent that develops when you are eating a diet high in fats and low in sugars. The fruity acid breath of the keto diet creates what is lovingly referred to as "keto mouth", and if you have ever smelled nail polish remover, you will know the smell. During the keto diet, you are fueling your body with almost all healthy fats, and virtually no glucose. When our bodies catabolize fat instead of glucose, we produce those helpful ketone bodies that will not stick to our fat cells and instead help promote that keto weight loss everyone looks for. However, our body's preferred source of energy is definitely not fatty acids, and the backup of ketone bodies in our bloodstream has more than a few negative effects.

Remember that a ketone body is made up of three main "ingredients", or chemical components: beta-hydroxybutyrate, acetone, and acetoacetate. Any reader who has ever gotten a full set of acrylic nails put on will recognize the ingredient "acetone" as the pungent-smelling chemical used to remove polish. This, unfortunately for dieters who have reached full-blown fat burning ketosis, is what your breath is going to smell like when your body is entirely switched over to metabolizing fats. Ketone bodies come out everywhere, from our urine to our sweat, and obviously, our breath. But you should not let this silly side effect discourage you from realizing what a good omen your bad breath actually is. Acetone present on your breath means that you have plenty of ketone bodies running through your bloodstream – an indicator that your body is functioning in full ketosis. In fact, some die-hard keto dieters use their bad breath as an indicator that they've entered into ketosis (but do not worry, they carry mints and gum afterward). Keto bad breath definitely is not the cutest symptom, but if your affliction is weight loss, it is certainly a symptom that you can manage in the name of trimming down.

The Keto "Brain Fog"

One of the strangest and more nuanced side effects of the keto diet is what participants commonly refer to as the "keto brain", a condition in which keto dieters experience intense mental fogginess. The neural cells and structures in your brain feed only on glucose in order to survive – which means that when you are eating a diet low in glucose, you do not have enough fuel for your brain. In the interim period between metabolizing glucose and metabolizing fat, your body tends to lack the twenty-five percent of its daily glucose intake that is required to run your brain. The good thing about the ketogenic brain fog is that once you have achieved ketosis, ketones can be used by your body to power your brain, and they are actually a more beneficial energy source – each ketone provides a more efficient energy source for your brain that takes *less* energy to breakdown into *more* usable energy. Although the keto brain fog can be hard to combat at first, you will find plenty of solutions to help you feel more awake and alert in the next section. Once you reach ketosis, your brain will begin to reap the benefits of a new overwhelming energy source, and most individuals tend to think that their thought processes are faster and clearer on a keto diet than they would be off one. If you think back to the types of diseases that the keto diet can manage, you might remember Alzheimer's, Parkinson's, and epilepsy. Eating a keto diet that fuels your brain with a more efficient and effective energy source *does* have a lasting and scientifically-proven effect on your neural health. You simply have to manage the aggravating symptoms of a metabolic shift in between a brain that functions decently and a brain that functions clearer than you might have imagined.

How to Kick Your Keto Slump

Getting over the hump of the carbohydrate flu that you might experience at the beginning of the keto diet is not hard, but it certainly is not self-explanatory. There are a few tried and true keto secrets that will help you amp up your energy levels on those days when you are craving a donut but can't eat carbs. The first, and probably most important, advice to kicking the keto slump is to learn how to make keto coffee. Yes, the keto diet has designed its own recipe for regular coffee, but you can trust the professionals when you try this delicious and fat-filled energy bomb. Keto coffee is very similar to the style of "bulletproof" coffee that blew up in popularity a few years ago. Bulletproof coffee was the first style of coffee to add thick, full-fat butter a cup of warm coffee in order to combat a low carbohydrate diet that just was not checking all the boxes. Keto coffee similarly consists of brewed black coffee, full-fat butter, and coconut oil or what is abbreviated as "MCT" oil, or medium-chain triglyceride oil. Medium-chain triglycerides are not entirely natural, although their components can be found in palm oil and coconut oil. Nonetheless, medium-chain triglycerides are incredibly healthy, doing everything from lowering our cholesterol to helping boost our energy and more effectively re-build torn muscles. Keto coffee is the perfect combination of the essential fats you need to ingest while eating keto and a boost of energy and healthful oils to start your day. If you aren't a big fan of coffee, you can try a keto hot-chocolate or a keto London fog by simply subbing in the ingredients. However, you might want to consider working in the element of caffeine, especially during your carbohydrate flu. The next best treatment you should consider taking to combat your negative side effects is what is called a "digestive enzyme". Digestive enzymes as a concept are present in our bodies already, but under certain conditions, we can accidentally strip them away or suddenly require more than we have. We need the help of chemical enzymes to help us with our digestion, and most of the time, our pancreas and liver do perfectly decent jobs of regulating these enzyme levels. However, when you begin eating a keto diet that is made up of mostly fat after a lifetime of eating sugars and carbs, your digestion will most likely struggle to compensate. Especially during your keto flu stage, digestive enzymes can help regulate your bowel movements and digestion to help combat some of the negative symptoms. Oftentimes a carb flu will also mean that your small and large intestines are unable to properly absorb your ingested nutrients, which means you might be wasting valuable energy and calories on a body that is not fit to digest. Adding digestive enzymes that you can take orally as tablets will help your stomach, pancreas, liver, and gallbladder do a better job of adapting to metabolizing fats without increasing the severity of your flu symptoms. Barring these techniques, there is one more trick that you can do to help you ease the uncomforting symptoms of the carbohydrate flu. But it is not a trick at all – it is something you should have been doing already, but especially during keto, it is time to take a hard look at your hydration to make sure that your body is in the best shape possible for your ketogenic reset.

Maintaining Your Hydration on a Keto Diet

Making sure that you are hydrated can be very tricky, especially in a modern corporate environment that demands we spend so much of our time sitting down. If you think that you might not drink enough water, you most likely do not. Almost everyone whose lifestyles is not immediately demanding of plenty of water is dehydrated right now. Per each day, one person on average should drink no less than half their body weight in ounces of water. The goal should be to drink between half your body weight and all of your body weight in ounces per day, but few of us make that. Hydration is important even if you are not on a restrictive diet that places your body under stress...and drinking water alone is scientifically proven to help you lose weight. Since so many of us are likely dehydrated, we are also likely holding on to toxin-riddled water weight around our midsections. When our bodies do not have a consistent enough supply of water, we hold on to the excess similar to storing glucose when we do not need it. Once you begin to rehydrate your systems, your body can finally purge itself of the stagnant and unhealthy water you've been holding onto. If drinking water on its own is this beneficial for your body, there's no reason you should not be doing so. In particular, while you are experiencing the symptoms of carbohydrate withdrawal, few things will be able to help your body wash out a headache like water can. Purchasing a sturdy water bottle at the beginning of your keto diet will serve you well in the long run – but there is one important nuance to consider before you start to drink hundreds of ounces of water per day.

Combating "Too Much Water"

Although we have established that almost all people are dehydrated in their daily lives, once you have started a keto diet, too much water can actually have a negative effect on your health. If you are planning to prepare for a few weeks before you begin a full keto diet, you will already be fully hydrated by the time you start. Our bodies need both water and something called electrolytes present in balanced quantities in order to regulate the amount of water inside, and outside, of our cells. Electrolytes, like salt, help our bodies by acting as electrical conductors when they are dissolved in water (if you are thinking about Gatorade – you are on the right track!). Sodium is the electrolyte found in salt, and it helps us regulate more than just the water distribution across our cells walls. Sodium is necessary to the function of our muscles and of our nerves, as well as to maintain our balance of potassium. Without a high enough sodium level, your body drops into a dangerous state of hyponatremia, a condition characterized by fatigue, dizziness, nausea, numbness, light-headedness, confusion, and in severe cases, seizures and an eventual comatose state. But a sodium deficiency doesn't just affect your stability and concentration - sodium, calcium, and potassium are all electrolytes, but it just so happens that sodium and potassium are intimately related to one another and to your body function. Sodium and potassium balance one another out in order to sustain your body's homeostasis, which is a long and technical word for your body's state of balance. Typically, our modern diets contain too much sodium, and if you are not used to eating fruits and vegetables regularly, your diet also probably lacks a large amount of potassium. Potassium regulates the sodium levels in our bloodstream, and typically is not dangerous in high levels. Regularly, if someone without a kidney disorder consumes too much potassium, the body will simply remove it as waste. If you have a kidney disorder, it will likely be harder for your body to filter out too much potassium, but that is a rare instance.

With this information in mind, think about what might happen when you shift to eating a keto diet that is packed full of potassium when you are not getting enough sodium. While you probably will not develop full hyperkalemia if you have well-functioning kidneys, you definitely will drop into a state of hyponatremia if you do not supplement your sodium intake. You can search out natural sources for sodium that work with a keto diet like eggs, whole milk, beets, celery, and various types of broth and bouillon. You can also find sodium in, surprise, salt! Adding more sodium to your ketogenic reset diet can be as simple as salting up your meals a little bit extra. If you want to make sure that you are getting enough sodium *without* adding extra salt to your entrees, you can purchase sodium tablets at any nutrition or vitamin store that you can take orally instead. Your keto diet will supply you with plenty of essential potassium to make sure you are functioning at your strongest, but sodium is necessary with the massive amount of water you will be flushing through your system every day.

Secret Keto Tricks and Tips

Sustaining Your Keto Lifestyle

The keto diet is not called a cult diet fad for no reason: people love it because it works, and it works well because there is an entire community of research supporting how to execute it properly. Science does not have to be scary, and a keto diet does not have to be intimidating with so many individuals who have paved the way for success before you. We are going to take a moment to talk in-depth about some tips and tricks that you can apply to your keto diet in order to maintain the most difficult aspects of the routine. Success is easily achievable with keto, but if you aren't getting started with the right tools, you could miss out on incredible weight loss opportunities. Ketosis is also a delicate process to maintain, and if you aren't sure what can knock you out of that coveted state of weight loss, you could fail before you've even gotten started. A keto lifestyle should not be about trying and failing to get healthy – it should be about learning all the ways that your body is naturally able to heal you. Up until now, you've learned enough of the science of the keto diet to take off on your own without any more advice. But, succeeding at something new is not just about learning the basic facts. Once you have all the insider knowledge on how to make keto work for you, there's no way that you will not be able to see results. If your ketogenic reset helps you discover new facts and knowledge that you think could benefit someone else, make sure to join the community of reviewers in the comments section to share your experience. The keto world is always looking for new and creative low-carb tricks, and our readers are one of the best sources for innovative knowledge. Once you've shared your story and let others know how the ketogenic reset has helped *you,* you might just learn a thing or two to implement into your diet. Speaking of diet...it is about time we talked a little bit more about everyone's favorite subject on a diet: the food!

Meal Preparation

Meal preparation in the twenty-first century might not directly refer to parents making their children's school lunches, but the concept behind both ideas is the same: saving time to offer healthier options. Meal preparation is a technique that was adopted by the bodybuilding community shortly after we gained more awareness into the unhealthy process of hydrogenating fats and oils. Busy fitness lovers who did not have enough time every day to pre-cook healthy and nutritious meals used to find themselves stuck in a fast food line that would immediately ruin their diet and not provide enough valuable nutrition to sustain their activity levels. Preparing your meals while you are eating on a strict diet will help you measure out your macronutrients properly, while also helping you measure out proper caloric and nutritional percentages for each meal. If you know that you are not going to be eating more than thirty grams of net carbohydrates per day, you can pay almost zero attention to what you are eating and still reach ketosis. Not only that, but ketosis is a state that is best reached through vigilant consistency; if each of your meals is the same, you will get there twice as fast. You will also be predisposed to maintain your state of ketosis longer if you know that your portions are measured to contain minimal carbs, high fat, and minimal protein. When it comes to weighing your meals and calculating your macronutrients, there is no easier and more effective way to make sure your macros are accounted for than through meal prep. But the benefits of a process will not do you any good if you do not know how to execute that process. Meal preparation is easy, but it certainly is not an easy amount of work if you aren't sure how to properly balance it. Once you learn how to meal prep properly, you will be able to calculate when scientifically, and for how long, your body can run effective ketosis for weight loss.

How to Meal Prep

Meal preparation doesn't really have a set of traditional rules, but there are a few guidelines that most of the meal preparation community tend to follow because they are effective. Most of the time, meal preppers will focus on making either their lunches and dinners or breakfasts and dinners for the week ahead, grocery shopping and cooking on the weekend before the work week gets in the way. By freeing up some of your time to focus on cooking healthy balanced meals, you might also free up time to make more mid-week gym sessions. The benefits of meal preparation are endless, but you have to make sure that your timing and organization are well primed for a long day of cooking. Make a list before you grocery shop with all the ingredients you need for you keto lunches and dinners, portioned out to three or four times the regular serving size for one person. When you are meal prepping, you want to decide whether you are going to cook meals for each weekday or just Monday through Thursday. On a keto diet, there are plenty of delicious options that you can order at a restaurant, so many dieters tend to meal prep for the workweek only to enjoy the weekend. Before you jump into cooking two meals each Sunday, start by preparing your dinners for four nights, and a few easy snacks. Meal prepping is all about supplies, so you will want to make sure that you have a clean kitchen stocked with clean pans, skillets, cooking utensils, and Tupperware. Using

Tupperware to store and keep your prepared meals will help you use your eyesight to confirm that one portion is not large than another – and matching Tupperware are a sure-fire way to ensure this happens. Be sure to take advantage of both your refrigerator and your freezer, because meals tend to take up a decent amount of space. Try and time out your cooking steps so that you can multi-task, which means paying attention to longer steps in one recipe that can simmer, sauté, or soak while you move on to your next recipe. It sounds like a harder task than it actually is because most keto meals do not require too many steps to make. Once you get the hang of meal prepping your entrees, it is always a good idea to think about smoothies, protein shakes, and on-the-go "fat bombs" that you can keep with you for snacks and in between meals. Although a low carbohydrate diet will tend to keep you feeling fuller for longer (something that a state of ketosis can also trigger), you want to make sure that you do not get caught without a snack when you are hungry. Keto "fat bombs" are snacks that are high in coconut oil, whole full fats, and healthy monounsaturated ingredients to make sure that you are always working towards a state of ketosis. They are a great snack to meal prep, and an easy way to get used to making your diet staples ahead of time. When it comes to tracking your macronutrients, there is no better time to use a food scale than when you are meal prepping. Food scales are the much more enjoyable counterpart to a weight scale, and they'll help you measure out how much of each macronutrient you have included in each portion of each meal – necessary information to your calorie deficit, as well. After you have meal prepped an entire batch of three or four serving entrees, you will want to measure your entire meal (all portions) together on your food scale. If you are in the market for new Tupperware, you might want to take a look at large plastic containers as well – these are necessary for holding all your ingredients on top of the scale at the same time. Once you have weighed your meal, enter your ingredient quantities into any fitness app or online calculator that can tell you how many calories, grams of carbohydrates, grams of protein, and grams of fat each one contains. Using this information, it is just a few quick math steps to work out the macronutrient percentages in each of your servings, as well as your caloric content. Since you prepared the meals yourself, you can also be sure that none of your natural oils or fats have been tampered with; they will all be monounsaturated, and will all have been cooked without added sugars. The key to meal prep is a commitment, but if you are already committed to a ketogenic lifestyle reset, you are already most of the way there. Plus, meal prepping is not just a concept for the fitness community. Plenty of large families with lots of mouths to feed and busy professionals looking to keep weight off without effort meal prep to achieve their goals. Implementing a process like meal prep into your lifestyle can only benefit your ketogenic diet, and you will be surprised how much more free time, and less stress, you will have once you learn.

Difference Between Low Carb And Keto Diets

Low carb diets have been ascending in ubiquity without any indications of dropping off. This isn't astounding when you consider the achievement of thousands of low carb calorie dieters who have quickly shed pounds and kept it off while improving their general wellbeing in the meantime.

Indeed, even the present literature underpins the viability of low carb diet for weight reduction and health improvement. Besides, numerous examinations additionally demonstrate that carb restriction can be utilized to help the treatment of conditions that low-fat diet may exacerbate.

Shockingly, in the event that you attempt to make sense of the best low-carb approach, you will be overpowered with one-sided and clashing data. A few sites guarantee that the keto diet is the best low carb diet since you get the advantages of ketosis and low-carb dieting concurrently, while others trust an increasingly permissive low-carb diet is the best approach in light of the fact that keto is excessively prohibitive and hazardous.

What information would it be a good idea for us to trust? All things considered, it relies upon the individual.

The initial step to understanding what diet may work best for you is understanding the contrast between a low carb diet and the ketogenic diet. After we sort out the specialized contrasts, we will look at that points burrow through the examination to enable you to disentangle what might be ideal for you.

The Low Carb Diet versus the Ketogenic Diet – The Technical Differences

Basically, a ketogenic diet or "keto diet" is a low-carb diet, yet not all low-carb diets are ketogenic diets.

The essential objective of the keto diet is to enable you to accomplish and continue dietary ketosis - a metabolic express what happens when the body reliably delivers and uses ketones for fuel. Limiting carbs underneath thirty-five grams for each day is generally all you have to do to enter and continue ketosis.

Regardless of whether you are on a keto diet or not can undoubtedly be replied by estimating your blood ketone levels. Are your ketone levels at 0.5 mmol/L or higher subsequent to executing the keto diet for a week or something like that? This shows you are really on the keto diet while any estimation lower than 0.5 mmol/L, in fact, implies that you are on a low carb diet, not a keto diet.

Lamentably, a similarly exact meaning of what a "low carb diet" is does not exist. Indeed, even the research literature doesn't appear to have a conclusive answer that enables us to interpret a low carb diet from a higher carb diet.

A few examinations characterize low-carb diet that limits carbs underneath 20% of calories while different investigations group it as a diet that comprises of under 45% carbs. The main thing that a great many people appear to concur on is the idea of driving the low-carb diet: to decrease carb admission by removing carbonic foods.

All the more explicitly, most low carb diets limit foods high in effectively edible carbs (e.g., sugar, bread, pasta, juice, soft drink) and supplant them with nourishments containing a higher level of fats and moderate protein (e.g., meat, poultry, fish, shellfish, eggs, cheddar, nuts, and seeds) and different nourishments low in carbs (e.g., non-bland vegetables, for example, spinach, kale, chard and broccoli), albeit different vegetables and natural products (particularly berries) are frequently permitted. The confinement of starches and certain nutritional categories fluctuate between the distinctive low carbohydrate diets.

A Brief Overview of the Most Popular Low Carb Diets

Because of its straightforward idea, the low carb diet can be drawn closer in a wide range of ways, some of which have turned out to be exceedingly mainstream over the previous decade. To show the wide scope of potential outcomes with regards to cutting carbs, how about we investigate the popular low carb diets:

A Typical Low-Carb Diet

The average low-carb diet does not have a fixed definition. This diet will, in general, be lower in carbs, and higher in protein than a commonplace "Western" diet.

This sort of low-carb diet is normally founded on meats, fish, eggs, nuts, seeds, vegetables, natural products, and sound fats. It limits the admission of high-carb foods like grains, potatoes, sugary beverages, and high-sugar prepared nourishments.

By changing to this dietary methodology from a higher-carb, westernized diet, the vast majority will get in shape and improve their health.

The Atkins Diet

The Atkins diet is a standout amongst the best known low-carb diet plans. This diet includes decreasing all high-carb nourishments while eating as much protein and fat as wanted.

The conventional Atkins diet consists of four stages:

Stage 1 – Induction: Eat under 20 grams of carbs every day for about fourteen days. This is fundamentally the same as a severe ketogenic diet.

Stage 2 – Balancing: Slowly include progressively nuts, low-carb vegetables, and organic products to your eating routine.

Stage 3 – Fine-tuning: When you draw nearer to your objective weight, include more carbs until weight reduction turns out to be slower.

Stage 4 – Maintenance: Once you've achieved your objective, eat the same number of solid carbs as your body endures without recovering the weight you lost.

The Atkins diet is all around explored and has been demonstrated to be both sheltered and viable for some individuals.

Eco-Atkins

The Eco-Atkins diet is essentially a veggie-lover rendition of the Atkins diet for those that need to cut carbs without eating such a significant number of animal products. It centers around plant foods and fixings that are high in protein as well as fat, for example, seitan, soy, nuts, and plant-based oils.

Because of the emphasis on plant foods, it is somewhat higher in carbs than an ordinary Atkins diet, yet at the same time much lower than an average veggie lover diet.

There aren't numerous investigations on this specific form of a low-carb diet. However, it seems to be sheltered and successful for weight reduction and improving a few parts of wellbeing.

A Low-Carb, Paleo Diet

The Paleo diet is, at present, a standout amongst the most famous dietary methodologies. This diet includes eating nourishments that were likely accessible in the paleolithic time and constraining the admission of foods that ended up well known after the farming and modern upheavals.

A Paleo diet doesn't concentrate on limiting carbs, yet since it removes a considerable lot of the most well-known foods we eat today, it normally is lower in carbs. The standard paleo diet wipes out handled foods, included sugar, grains, vegetables, and dairy products, and spotlights on top-notch meats, fish, vegetables, natural products, and a few nuts and seeds.

A few little examinations are demonstrating that a Paleo diet can cause weight reduction, a decrease in blood sugars and improved hazard factors for coronary illness, like what happens because of following other low carb abstains from food.

Numerous other prevalent adaptations of the Paleo diet exist, for example, the basic outline and the ideal healthy diet.

A Scandinavian Low Carb, High-Fat Diet (LCHF)

Sweden was one of the primary nations to condemn the belittling of fat and greet it wholeheartedly. The basic role of the diet is to initiate weight reduction and forestall unending illnesses by decreasing carbs and expanding fats.

The Scandinavian low carb, high-fat diet concentrates more on food quality and is more prohibitive than the average low-carb diet.

For instance, dietary staples are:

Grass-fed beef, field raised poultry and other fatty meats, fish and seafood's, full-fat dairy products, plant-based fats: Coconut and olive oil. Low carb veggies: Cauliflower, broccoli, cabbage, kale, collards, bok choy, spinach, and so forth. Also, berries, nuts, and seeds.

What's more, foods that ought to be kept away from on this eating routine are:

High-glycemic fruits, grains, starchy veggies, juices. Prepared or bundled nourishment/drinks with included sugar.

This diet is less severe than a significant number of the weight control plans on this rundown and might be one of the most advantageous too.

The Carnivore Diet (Zero Carb Diet)

The carnivore diet depends on the conviction that we don't need to bother with plant nourishments or dietary carbs to endure. A few defenders of this methodology imagine that the defensive components in plants are what cause numerous regular medical problems, so following a diet that comprises of every single animal products might be the best approach to ideal wellbeing.

There is no exploration to back up the proposed medical advantages of this dietary methodology. Indeed, most of the writing prompts against constraining plant admission and determining the vast majority of your calories from creature items, particularly since they are inadequate in significant supplements like nutrient C and fiber.

The Low-Carb Mediterranean Diet

The Mediterranean diet is mainstream, particularly among health experts and specialists, for its medical advantages. It includes choosing nourishments that were (apparently) devoured in Mediterranean nations during the prior part of the twentieth century. Therefore, the diet basically comprises of vegetables, natural products, nuts, seeds, vegetables, potatoes, full grains, bread, herbs, flavors, fish, and additional virgin olive oil.

Following quite a while of research on this dietary methodology, the Mediterranean diet has collected a lot of research support up its medical advantages.

A low-carb Mediterranean diet is essentially a Mediterranean diet that breaking points higher-carb foods like full grains, potatoes, and vegetables. It is like a normal low-carb diet, then again, actually it emphasizes progressively fatty fish rather than red meat, and all the more additional virgin olive oil rather than animal fat such as butter.

Since it favors fatty fish and olive oil, a low-carb Mediterranean diet might be preferred for coronary illness over other low-carb diets, in spite of the fact that this should be affirmed in studies.

Tim Ferriss' Slow Carb Diet

The Slow Carb diet was made in 2010 by writer and business visionary Tim Ferriss, who distributed the standards in his top-rated book "The 4-Hour Body."

The diet pursues these five basic standards:

Rule 1: Avoid prepared foods, bread, pasta, and anything made with refined flour.

Rule 2: Eat a similar couple of sound dinners over and again

Rule 3: Don't drink calories (aside from several glasses of red wine every night, whenever liked)

Rule 4: Don't eat fruits

Rule 5: Have a cheat day where you can eat anything you'd like

The greater part of calories on the low carb diet will come from:

Proteins: Grass-fed beef, poultry, pork, fish, seafood's and without lactose-free whey powder. Vegetables such as lentils, beans, chickpeas, and soybeans. Low-glycemic vegetables: Leafy greens, broccoli, cauliflower, kale, asparagus, peas, and other non-starchy veggies. Fats like Nuts, sans dairy half and half, macadamia oil, olive oil, and grape seed oil. Flavors: Salt, garlic salt and herbs.

With the infrequent, curds are the main dairy product permitted.

Red wine is the main beverage with calories permitted. In spite of the fact that there has been no exploration done on this diet, it appears to advance comparative weight reduction and wellbeing enhancements. This diet might be a decent choice for the individuals who would prefer not to surrender carb-rich nourishments totally.

Whole30 Diet

The Whole30 is a 30-day program which was made by games nutritionists Dallas Hartwig and Melissa Hartwig in 2009. It was made to take out conceivably risky foods for in any event 30 days and just eating nourishments that have wellbeing advancing impact for the vast majority.

To pursue this diet, you essentially focus on eating entire, low carb foods that aren't in the restricted classes and stay away from possibly unsafe elements for 30 days.

The nourishments you can eat on this diet include proteins such as meat, poultry, fish. Low carb veggies: Broccoli, spinach, tomatoes, peppers. Low-glycemic natural products: berries, kiwi, lemon. Common fats: Olive oil, coconut oil, avocado, ghee. 100% natural product juices

Explicit vegetables like green beans, sugar snap peas, and snow peas

Vinegar. Herbs and flavors.

The nourishments that you ought to dispose of totally for 30 days includes sugar, genuine, or fake. No maple syrup, nectar, agave nectar, coconut sugar, and other included sugars. Grains: Wheat, rye, grain, oats, corn, rice, millet, bulgur, sorghum, grew grains, all without gluten oats, grain, germ, and starch. Vegetables: Beans of different types, peas, chickpeas, lentils, peanuts, nutty spread, and all types of soy. Dairy: cow, goat or sheep results, for example, milk, cream, cheddar, kefir, yogurt, acrid cream, dessert, or solidified yogurt.

Prepared treats and low-quality nourishment.

When these nourishments are killed from the diet for 30 days, the individual can gradually add them back in to perceive how it influences their wellbeing and vitality levels. On the off chance that the nourishment is risky for the individual in any capacity, at that point, it is ideal to keep it out of the diet totally. Then again, foods that are all around endured might be allowed with some restraint.

No investigation has been done on this diet explicitly. However, it has the possibility to improve by and large the health and help individuals get in shape. This dietary methodology may likewise be useful for those hoping to check whether they are delicate to foods that fall in the class of vegetables, dairy, and grains.

The Ketogenic Diet

The ketogenic diet is intended to keep carb utilization so low that the body goes into a metabolic state called ketosis.

At the point when carb admission is exceptionally low, insulin levels drop fundamentally, making an inward situation that animates the arrival of a lot of unsaturated fats from muscle versus fat stores. A great deal of these unsaturated fats are moved to the liver, where they might be transformed into ketones.

Ketones (otherwise called ketone bodies) are water-soluble atoms that can fuel most of the cells all through the body, including the greater part of the synapses'. On the off chance that the body is in ketosis for an all-inclusive timeframe, ketones will inevitably supply up to half of the body's basal vitality necessities and 70% of the mind's vitality needs. The glucose that is as yet required by the cerebrum and body will be delivered by the liver by means of a procedure called gluconeogenesis.

A ketogenic diet centers on high-protein and high-fat foods, while a few adaptations of keto endeavor to constrain the admission of high-protein nourishments with the goal that the protein won't diminish ketone levels. Carbs are commonly restricted to under 50 grams for each day. However, we prescribe beginning with 35 grams or less.

A regular ketogenic diet is alluded to as a "standard" ketogenic diet (SKD).

Nonetheless, there are different varieties that include deliberately adding carbs to fuel high-power work out: Directed Ketogenic Diet (TKD) – Add modest quantities of carbs around high-force exercises.

Recurrent Ketogenic Diet (CKD) – Eat a ketogenic diet on most days of the week yet change to a high-carb diet for 1–2 days every week.

The Bigger Picture – Which Low-Carb Diet is best for you?

As should be obvious, there are a wide cluster of varieties for the low-carb diet, and we haven't started to expose what is conceivable.

Each diet can be balanced interminably. The keto diet, for instance, can likewise be changed over into a without dairy, veggie-lover, or vegan diet that advances ketosis.

This implies you can utilize the ideas from these low-carb diets to plan a diet that encourages you to accomplish your body creation objectives and improve your wellbeing in the meantime. Be that as it may, doing this expects us to delve further into the examination on keto and low carb diets to comprehend the standards behind their adequacy.

Low-Carb versus Keto – Which One is Better for Weight Loss?

I still can't seem to discover any examination looking at a non-keto, low carb diet (that doesn't incite continued ketosis) to a keto diet, so it will be hard to make direct correlations with respect to weight reduction. Hypothetically, it is enticing to imagine that keto diets are better since they limit carbs more than most low-carb diet.

Notwithstanding, the ebb and flow research literature doesn't bolster this conviction. Meta-investigations that analyze the keto diet (<50 grams of carbs every day) with low-fat diet and low-carb diet (<45% of calories originating from carbs) with low-fat diet show just a slight weight reduction advantage for cutting carbs (about 2 pounds of additional weight reduction following a half year or more contrasted with a low-fat diet).

As it were, these three diets – keto, low-carb, and low-fat – would all be able to enable us to lose a comparative amount of weight following a half year. This additionally recommends there may not be a discernible contrast in weight reduction results between non-keto, low-carb diets, and extremely low carb, keto diet.

Albeit no top-notch information exists that can enable us to make an immediate examination between keto diet and less prohibitive low-carb diet. The present writing proposes that carb utilization may not be the most significant variable with regards to getting more fit.

This hypothesis increases further help when we incorporate the information from an ongoing meta-examination of controlled encouraging preliminaries that coordinated protein and calorie utilization while shifting the carb and fat food of the diet. Investigating studies led as such gives us the most precise approach to unravel the contrasts between cutting carbs and cutting fat with everything else coordinated.

True to form from the consequences of the meta-investigations examined prior, the analysts found no huge contrast between low-carb and low-fat weight control plans when calorie and protein admission were equivalents for each gathering. In this way, the present information demonstrates that keeping up a caloric shortage is the way to weight reduction, not carb limitation.

All things considered, low-carb diets do appear to give us a genuine favorable position over higher-carb, lower-fat weight control plans.

All the more explicitly, there are two key rules that clarify why cutting carbs work so well for weight reduction:

By confining carbs, you normally increment your utilization of high-fat, protein-thick, and fiber-rich foods. These foods support satiety levels in the short-

and long haul, which makes you eat fewer calories than previously.

By confining carbs, you are wiping out; basically, all calorically-thick handled foods from your diet. These foods are commonly so acceptable that they cause us to expend such a large number of calories and increase fat.

At the end of the day, by following a low carb diet, we will, in general, expend fewer calories than expected and get in shape. This may clarify why low carb and keto appear to give comparative measures of weight reduction (when contrasted with low-fat diet).

Could Keto Give Us Slight Fat Loss Advantage?

In any case, it is additionally conceivable that keto diet can build satiety and weight reduction more than a non-keto, low-carb diet on the grounds that by cutting carbs low enough we can use the advantages of a low-carb diet alongside the craving smothering properties of ketones.

How much additional weight reduction somebody can get from being in ketosis is misty. Research presently can't seem to legitimately investigate the impact that ketones can have on our calorie utilization and body arrangement.

In summary, the information propose that non-keto, low-carb diets, and keto diets lead to comparative measures of weight reduction. Regardless of whether future research demonstrates that keto builds weight reduction more than other low-carb diets. People question the distinction will be critical enough to crown the keto diet as the best eating routine for weight reduction for everybody.

Nonetheless, we should recall that weight reduction isn't the main thing we ought to be centered around when settling on diet choices. The most significant variable to consider, as a matter of first importance, is the manner by which your diet and way of life influence your general health.

Low Carb versus Keto – Short-Term Health Effects

How about we dunk our toes into the pool of health by outlining the present information on low-carb diets and how they influence distinctive wellbeing conditions and biomarkers of wellbeing. Probably the most well-considered and surely understood biomarkers are triglycerides, cholesterol, glucose, A1c, and circulatory strain, and every one of them have been found to improve altogether because of diet (for the vast majority).

Research additionally demonstrates that low carb diets can help individuals with the accompanying conditions of type 2 diabetes, type 1 diabetes, hypertension, high blood sugar levels, coronary illness, polycystic ovary syndrome, fatty liver disease, and acne.

Some proof proposes that a keto diet might be more viable than a less-prohibitive low carb diet at helping patients with diabetes, high glucose levels, hypertension, fatty liver sickness, and polycystic ovary disorder.

Moreover, keto diets have been found to help patients who have Alzheimer, Parkinson, Epilepsy, chemical imbalance spectrum disorder, gout, and cancer.

Dietary ketosis is the mystery fixing behind the beneficial outcomes that keto can have on the neurological issue recorded above, gout, and numerous kinds of cancer.

To put it plainly, the keto diet might be more useful and more beneficial than a less-prohibitive low carb diet on the off chance that you have one of the conditions recorded previously. So, carb utilization plays a significant job in our wellbeing (mostly by assisting with hormonal guideline and supplanting overabundance calories from fat). Along these lines, a few people may encounter an exacerbating of their health because of following a keto diet.

The most effective method to know whether a Keto Diet is Healthy for You

In spite of the fact that carbs aren't fundamental, it is conceivable to experience issues with your cholesterol levels, Thyroid hormone levels because of following a keto diet.

In the event that the keto diet isn't improving your general wellbeing, at that point, it might be ideal to build your carb utilization until your applicable biomarkers improve (cholesterol levels, thyroid hormone levels, and so on.). In any case, this doesn't mean you should simply begin eating whatever food is accessible on the grounds that this will aggravate your health status even.

Rather, it is ideal to pursue a whole food-based, low-carb diets like the Paleo diet or a low-to-direct carb Mediterranean diet. Following a month or so of following your new methodology, it might be ideal to get another blood test to perceive how your biomarkers are getting along

Low-Carb versus Keto Diet – Long-Term Health and Longevity

A 2018 observational investigation and meta-examination was as of late distributed in the Lancet on the subject of carb utilization and mortality chance, and numerous news outlets spun the information in a manner the made low carb diet look deadly. Be that as it may, when we take a gander at all of the information from the first examination, a considerably more nuanced example unfurls.

By and large, it seems conceivable that a low carb diet prompts a diminished life expectancy, however just when it infers the vast majority of its calories from creature items (i.e., creature fats, meat, and prepared meats). In any case, when low carb diets comprise of more plant-based foods, for example, vegetables, nuts, vegetables, and grains, mortality risks diminishes essentially.

At the end of the day, a low-carb, carnivore type diet is likely not useful for the health for the vast majority in the long haul, and a plant-based, low-carb diet may decrease our mortality risk in excess of a moderate carb diet (the one diet that numerous news stories guarantee to be most beneficial).

All things considered, figuring out what the best diet is for long haul wellbeing relies upon the person. By and large, supplanting high-carb foods and prepared meats with more plant-based whole foods is a decent spot to begin.

When the diet begins to incline toward all the more whole food and less prepared nourishments, the health and body system will in general improve. Regardless of whether you get progressively exacting with carb utilization relies upon how well you do with wholesome ketosis and the end result for your wellbeing as you decline carbs and increment fat and protein.

As we found before, a few people may charge better with a diet that doesn't expand fat utilization and abate carb consumption so much, while others may flourish when they are in nourishing ketosis.

Low-Carb versus Keto – Which One is Easier to Follow

A standout amongst the most significant dietary rules that a large number of us disregard is the means by which simple is to pursue. A large portion of us can get spurred for transient weight reduction, yet will you have the order to continue your dietary methodology for longer than a couple of months?

With regards to improving your wellbeing and getting thinner, consistency is vital. All the more explicitly, we should pursue a diet that can reliably enable us to accomplish our objectives and continue our outcomes without bouncing back.

As it were, in the event that you can't transform your dietary methodology into your new long haul way of life, at that point it is ideal to stay away from it.

For the vast majority, the more prohibitive a diet is, the harder it will be to support for longer timeframes. This implies it might be increasingly hard for huge numbers of us to stay with the keto diet contrasted with a non-keto, low-carb diet.

When you are picking a dietary methodology, you should be totally fair with yourself. Remember to consider elements like what your family eats, your nourishment condition, your way of life, and your present habits.

Do you figure you could stay with this diet without bouncing back to old habits months after the fact? If not, what do you want to do to enable you to accomplish and support your outcomes without it being a steady battle?

Need assistance? Here are a few methodologies that can make your outcomes simpler to accomplish and support: Attempt an alternate diet that fits better with your way of life. Take a stab at combining various weight control plans (e.g., switch among Keto and a Paleo diet at regular intervals). Also, try to utilize little plates/parcel sizes to eat the measure of food you eat at every feast. Expel every single bad food from your home and never get them again. Moreover, make sure to have solid food choices promptly accessible and make bad foods a lot harder to accomplish and devour. Increase your activity levels for the duration of the day (e.g., utilize a standing work area, take strolls, do light stretches, take move breaks). In addition, Track your calorie consumption with a calorie following application. Have a sound nibble with you while you are making a course for shield you from halting for cheap food. Also, Have a go at skipping breakfast (irregular fasting).

On the off chance that you don't know what to attempt, move your considerations to a long haul point of view. Which procedure can you effectively make a piece of your way of life? Out it a go after in any event a month and assess your outcomes to check whether you need to keep utilizing it, add another system to it, or trial with something different.

What's more, dependably recollect that steady minded individuals will win in the end, particularly with regards to weight reduction and wellbeing advancement. The individuals who get thinner at a delicate pace of 1 to 2 pounds for each week are substantially more prone to keep it off than the individuals who get more fit at a lot quicker rate.

As we talked about previously, the way to shedding pounds is continuing a calorie shortfall. Being in ketosis and limiting carbs can help, yet in the event that you continually battle with these two things, at that point you may need to pursue a less prohibitive eating routine that encourages you to keep up a calorie shortage and improve wellbeing by utilizing different techniques.

Non-Keto, Low Carb Diets versus the Keto Diet – Which One is Better Overall?

Is keto the better of the low-carb class? Is it accurate to say that one low-carb diet superior to the others? Similarly, as with most health-related inquiries, the most exact answer is "it depends." Every famous assortment of the low-carb diet can possibly improve wellbeing and help individuals get thinner. However, everyone influences every individual in an unexpected way.

The keto diet, for instance, might be the best diet for individuals who react well to it from both an emotional (i.e., improved feeling of prosperity) and goal (i.e., improved biomarkers and body arrangement) point of view. Additionally, the wealth of ketones that we produce when following this dietary methodology may animate more weight reduction, upgrade intellectual capacity, and improve different parts of wellbeing. Keto may likewise be the best diet for patients who have epilepsy, Parkinson's ailment, Alzheimer's ailment, and a few sorts of cancer.

Then again, non-keto, low-carb diets might be an extraordinary path for individuals to improve their general wellbeing and body creation without stressing over their ketone levels. Since low-carb diets support additionally satisfying foods (i.e., foods that are high in fiber, fat, or potentially protein), individuals that pursue these diets will, in general, feel fuller, eat fewer calories, and shed pounds. A less prohibitive low-carb diet will, in general, be significantly more reasonable as a long haul way of life and more advantageous for the individuals who battle with elevated cholesterol levels, adrenal issues, as well as thyroid issues.

What might work best for you?

As a rule, on the off chance that you choose to diminish carb utilization in any way, shape or form, the ebb, and flow research demonstrates that a great many people will decrease their mortality chance and improve generally speaking wellbeing by subbing out exceptionally foods and animal products for low-carb, negligibly prepared plant nourishments.

It is likewise imperative to think about how reliable you can be with your diet. Confused weight control plans that you can't imagine yourself following for longer than a couple of months are not by any means worth attempting. The best strategy to get more slender, have more vitality, improve mental center, and upgrade by and large wellbeing is to receive a more beneficial way of life that you can keep up uncertainly.

The initial step to embracing a solid way of life is picking a diet that is supported by research to give the advantages it asserts and alter your methodology from that point. To enable you to evaluate what diet, to begin with, here are probably the most significant characteristics of a solid eating routine: It is an open and reasonable way of life change for you. It has been experimentally demonstrated to give the advantages that you are searching for. Also, It gives you a wide assortment of micronutrients from a few nutrition classes. In addition, It utilizes straightforward nourishment decides that you can pursue.

As you begin making acclimations to your eating routine and way of life, ensure you are monitoring these factors: How you feel, the adjustments in your body structure and the essential biomarkers.

At the point when everyone is inclining the correct way, you will realize that you are settling on sound diet and way of life decisions for you.

The Best Lifestyle Complements to a Keto Diet

Intermittent Fasting

The Benefits of Intermittent Fasting

If you have skipped previous sections that are triggering to individuals with disordered eating or neurotic tendencies, you might want to skip this section as well. Although intermittent fasting is an entirely scientific and useful way to manage your health, the science is still out on whether or not fasting has a negative effect on certain mental states. You should also take into consideration that intermittent fasting, as well as fasting of any kind, is dangerous for individuals with heart conditions. You should always consult your general practitioner before committing to a routine that drastically effects your normal biological processes.

Intermittent fasting is not a new concept in nutritional spheres, but it has historically been used to treat very specific disorders or to target weight loss in individuals with dangerous levels of obesity. However, intermittent fasting has incredible metabolic benefits if you perform it under the correct healthy guidelines. Intermittent fasting works similarly to a cleanse or a detox, derived from the theory that your body tends to become blocked or clogged by harmful bi-products when we are not facilitating effective disposal methods. When you eat a diet that is too high in carbohydrates, processed grains, and hydrogenated fats and oils, your digestive system is used to materials that offer little nutritional value and run right through your system. Carbs and processed ingredients are very easy for our bodies to break down, but they are also full of harmful sugars. When your body *can* easily digest something, it will – and if you are digesting processed foods, you are going to absorb those sugars just as quickly as you can digest. Processed foods therefore almost always cause unhealthy spikes in your blood sugar, and if your body is used to consuming plenty of daily sugars, your bloodstream is going to be blocked and clogged with glucose. One of the benefits of intermittent fasting is allowing your body to re-regulate your blood glucose levels back to normal numbers, which lowers your blood pressure and calms inflammation. As this happens towards the beginning of a fast, your digestion also slows down and begins to enter that starvation phase that so makes so many keto dieters unduly nervous. When you restrict your eating, it actually retrains your digestive tract to more effectively absorb the nutrients that you are eating – and more effectively process the nutrients you have already stored. When your body is in a state of fasting, your system sends out various hormonal signals that decrease your insulin levels in order to release tough stores of glycogen. If your insulin levels are lower than normal already, as they are during a keto diet, your body will not have to do all that much work in order to access your stored fat. Access to stored fat means the ability to burn your stored fat, and this is why intermittent fasting tends to promote weight loss. However, remember what happens when you eat meals that contain glucose when you do not have a hefty enough supply of insulin. Diets that are high in carbohydrates do not work well when paired with intermittent fasting because your fuel source is mostly glucose. A rapid intake of sugar after or during a fast will inevitably cause a large and unhealthy spike in your blood sugar. On a ketogenic reset diet, you will be eating such little glucose that your blood sugar will be much less likely to spike. Not to mention fibrous vegetables and fruits and high fat content ingredients take a long time for our system to digest, which already predisposes our blood sugar to rise at a slow and consistent rate. Intermittent fasting, when paired with a keto diet, is incredibly beneficial to stimulate your weight loss without sending your body into too much distress. But that is not the only reason keto dieters tend to pair fasting with a high fat diet; if you think back to the bi-products that the keto diet produces, you might remember that full ketosis sends a decent amount of ketone bodies into your bloodstream. Intermittent fasting on a keto diet helps you to regulate your ketone levels while also boosting your energy levels and fighting off the pesky symptoms of the carbohydrate flu.

Why Intermittent Fasting is Essential for a Keto Diet

Intermittent fasting is not just a helpful tool that you can use to lose weight. When you are eating on a ketogenic diet, you are likely going to experience some uncomfortable symptoms during the first few weeks – and if you keep in mind that you cannot *always* eat keto, you might have more than a few sets of "first weeks". The keto diet should never be extremely strenuous for your body if you are taking the right precautions, but many people will experience fatigue, brain fog, weakness, migraines, and sleep issues anyway. The state of ketosis that a ketogenic diet attempts to help you reach is actually very similar to the state of starvation that your body enters during a fast. When you aren't getting enough glucose, your body re-wires your system for fat metabolism, and you begin to produce those high energy ketones that will fuel your life processes. Fatigue, weakness, and brain fog are some of the most annoying side effects of the keto flu, but intermittent fasting helps you eliminate those symptoms in almost no time. If you choose to take on a twenty-four hour fast, you can sometimes see in improvement in your mental clarity, concentration, energy levels, and attitude within the same amount of time. And, if you are already fueling your body with a ketogenic diet, you will already be primed and ready to promote and sustain the ketosis that intermittent fasting will help you achieve. You obviously never have to take on an intermittent fast of any kind if you feel uncomfortable, but there are plenty of workable methods of fasting that will benefit any type of lifestyle. Fasting and the keto diet are a perfect pair, and if you are ready to see just how much weight you can lose on the keto diet with intermittent fasting, let's take a closer look at how you can get there.

Methods of Intermittent Fasting

There are many different methods for intermittent fasting, from two-day long stints without any sustenance to sixteen-hour breaks between meals. Finding the best intermittent fasting method for you is closely related to how your body likes to eat, and *when* your body likes to eat. If you often find yourself nauseous first thing the morning and unable to eat breakfast, you might want to consider a sixteen-hour fast that extends through your nighttime break in eating into mid-morning the next day. If you are more likely to be the type of person who wakes up starving, you might want to avoid this method of fasting, and instead opt for doing a caloric fast that simply limits your intake, instead of eliminating it. The most popular method of fasting in the keto community tends to be the overnight sixteen to eight ratio, where you spend sixteen hours fasting including your sleep and eat during an eight-hour window in the middle of the day between noon and eight p.m. Although some individuals who eat on the keto diet chose to fast for two days (twenty-four hours) straight once or twice a week, this is a difficult method if you do not think you can manage to wait from one meal one day to that same meal the next day to eat. Effective twenty-four hour fasts usually begin after you finish dinner the first night and then end when you *begin* to eat your dinner at the same time you *finished* your dinner the night before. If you have a busy day ahead of your, this might be an ideal fast for a distracted mind. If you do not want to stop eating entirely, but you still want to reap the benefits of an intermittent fasting schedule, you can eat on a keto fast that restricts your calories only. For two days each week that are not back to back, this style of fasting limits your caloric intake to only five hundred calories for smaller individuals and six hundred calories for larger individuals. During each of the other five days of the week, you should make sure to eat your full fifteen hundred to twenty-five hundred calorie diet – and you should eat it at the exact same time. This type of fast tends to be less effective if you eat your meals sporadically, so you need to make sure that you are consistent with your meal times and snack times. Like any relatively drastic system of dieting, if you feel any adverse side effects during any regime of intermittent fasting, you should consult a medical professional before slowly introducing liquids and solid foods back into your diet.

The Keto "Fat Fast"

In case you were getting a little hungry thinking about all the foods that you cannot eat during an intermittent fast, let's talk instead about what's called the keto "fat fast" – the total opposite of a real fast. Keto fat fasts can be used in one of two ways, and both can have an incredible impact on your ketosis and your weight loss. During a fat fast, you will want to aim to eat the same amount of calories that you always do – except you will want to get ninety to one-hundred percent of them from fats only. Yes, it's a lot of fat, and a lot of fatty acids to pump into your system. However, fat fasts are used in healthy ways that do not overwhelm your system. Many keto dieters who eat a cyclical keto program will use a fat fast to ramp up their fatty acid content and jump-start their ketosis at the full-time level they left off. You can also use a fat fast to compensate for a day of eating too many carbohydrates, too much protein, or too much processed sugar. A fat fast will help your body quickly un-do the damage caused by an unbalanced diet, and the infusion of almost 100% dietary fat will never do anything but help you have a more successful bought of ketosis. Most fat fasts do not last longer than a few days (often a maximum of five), and you should take note that a drastically unbalanced form of eating like this shouldn't be something that you take on frequently. The second way that many keto dieters use a fat fast is to stimulate stubborn weight loss. Occasionally, when an individual has been eating a keto diet for more than month or so, their bodies become adjusted to the lifestyle, and they stop losing weight. Sometimes, your body can reach a sort of "plateau" on the keto diet when you strip away all your stored fats but aren't at enough of a deficit in your diet or fitness routine to continue stimulating weight loss. A fat fast will jolt your body into a state of effective and efficient short-term ketosis, and they are a tried and true method to help reset your metabolism if you've gotten too used to eating a keto diet.

How to Exercise During an Intermittent Fast

It is not always obvious on the keto diet when the best times are to exercise, and especially if you are experiencing the side effects of the keto flu or struggling to handle cravings during a fast, you might have no desire to work out. There are a few key exercises you can do though, particularly during an intermittent fasting period that will actually help you feel better if you can believe that. Stimulating our muscles, boosting circulation, and raising your heart rate while feeling crummy on keto can help your body tap into sealed energy stores, metabolize nutrients faster, and recover quickly. But remember – you are still eating on a keto diet, and so you will still be limited to exercises that do not raise your heart rate too high, and will not make you breathe too hard. On an intermittent fast, the best exercises are the ones that go well with your keto diet: yoga and Pilates, strength and flexibility exercises, and bodyweight routines. You should also, however, pay attention to the type of fast that you have chosen to conduct. If you are fasting overnight, it is generally a good idea to do any cardio activities when your stomach is empty first thing in the morning. You have to worry a little bit less about planning your meal times and workouts if you have chosen to eat a fast the only limits your calorie intake, instead of eliminating it. On the other side of that coin, if you've decided to complete a twenty-four hour fast, you might want to consider working out towards the beginning and doing a restorative activity towards the end of your fast to keep your circulation flowing and your muscles from getting too tense. The most important thing about exercising on an intermittent fast in combination with the keto diet is that you must listen to your body. If you feel too dehydrated, or the opposite, too sodium-depleted, it is a good idea to consider taking a few days off the gym while you are trying to fast. After all, the point of a fast in the first place is to stimulate ketosis and promote your weight loss, and if you are already going to lose a few pounds during a fast, it is probably okay to take a break.

Why the Keto Diet Itself Should Be Intermittent

One of the most left-out details about the ketogenic diet in most keto guide books is that you cannot simply start eating keto and then never stop. Although keto is incredibly effective as a short-term diet, placing your body in ketosis for longer than a few weeks can be very damaging to your health. While some dieters claim that you can become what is called "keto-adapted", there's no healthy way for you to force your body to do something it doesn't naturally enjoy doing. Luckily, there are plenty of ways to alternate between eating keto and eating a more regularly carbohydrate-filled diet to modulate the negative effects of ketones in your blood. The keto diet also needs to be eaten on and off in order to make sure that you do not over-tax your system. Remember the negative effects that ketosis can have on your body? Besides lacking the essential glucose that your brain prefers to use as a fuel source, a keto diet can cause both diarrhea and constipation, gall stones, mental fogginess, and incredibly low energy levels. Sometimes, depending on your body type and lifestyle, these symptoms can be more difficult to manage while you are in ketosis. Thankfully, ketosis is not a process that is going away any time soon, and it is incredibly easy for you to eat a keto diet that allows you the occasional carbohydrate-packed meal in order to balance out your homeostasis. One of the ways of balancing a keto diet with your personal lifestyle is something we have touched on before: carbo-loading for athletes. Eating a keto diet that offers you some flexibility is as simple as choosing a few days, or weeks, in which you eat a higher carb diet and work out a little bit extra. Ketosis is generally easy to enter once you've already gone through the process once, and so it is generally fairly easy to slide in and out of if you are maintaining your body. There is also a sneaky trick that the keto community developed in order to boost dieters back into ketosis quickly. If you do not like protein shakes, it might be time to think about smoothies. You can purchase and take something called "exogenous ketones" which are ingestible ketone bodies in a protein-powder form. Each serving will dose your body with extra ketones and pull you back into ketosis more quickly than if you'd been attempting to re-enter keto with your diet only. A ketogenic reset is all about finding the routine that works for your lifestyle because a sustainable diet will always promote more long-term weight loss than a diet that you struggle to commit to.

The Ketogenic Diet and Animal Products

Although the keto diet by itself is an incredibly

beneficial pattern of eating, sometimes you might find yourself wondering why you have not removed many of the processed and hydrogenated animal products that contain so many unhealthy materials. Many individuals that chose to eat a ketogenic diet also chose to eat a keto diet free of animal products, for many of the same reasons that they have chosen to eat keto in the first place. A keto diet focuses on fueling your body with whole, natural, healthy fats, instead of sugary carbohydrates, because of glucose fuels a mechanism that we do not want to trigger. However, carbohydrates tend to be packed full of chemically altered fats, sugars, and oils, and almost none of the fats found in processed animal products are un-hydrogenated. You do not have to support the animals to understand why a ketogenic diet that eliminates animal products alongside everything else is simply, well, logical. And as is the case with science and logic, it tends to follow that if you eat less unhealthy material, you will suffer fewer unhealthy consequences. Individuals who combine their ketogenic diets with a vegan or "pescetarian" mindset (the latter meaning a diet that allows you to eat seafood but no other animals products) will lose more pounds over a shorter amount of time than someone whose ketogenic diet includes possible hidden carbs, processed sugars, and unhealthy additives. Remember back to when we discussed monosaccharides and the healthy sugars that your body needs to function. Unhealthy sugars, called disaccharides, are only one step away from being beneficial for your body, but they just do not get close enough. Lactose is one of these types of disaccharides, and it is also known as "milk sugar". If you aren't entirely sure that your milk is lactose-free, then you could be consuming more glucose than you realize. Ketosis is hard enough to achieve when you are operating on a strict keto diet, but many people simply chose to make it easier on themselves by going vegan. One of the best recommendations for keto diet styles is a seafood-focused keto diet that allows you to eat fish, but either option will offer you nothing but benefits in combination with your keto diet.

Keto-Friendly Diet Swaps

Eating a ketogenic diet does not have to mean that you give up all your favorite foods – by now, you have seen the recipes and know what you are in for in the kitchen. But if you are used to a few necessary staples, like sugar in your morning coffee or chocolate cake for dessert, there are a few substitutions that you can make to enjoy your keto diet a little bit more. And for those of you who want to maximize your weight loss during ketosis, there are a few key supplements you will want to know in order to get the most bang for your keto buck. You already know that cauliflower can be used to make delicious imitation chicken wings and buffalo chicken bites, but cauliflower can also be a great substitute for rice and any sort of bread-like material. If you are wondering what "bread-like material" could mean, think of things like pizza crusts, flat tortilla rounds, and burrito bowls. The best thing about eating a ketogenic diet is that you are often forced to get creative with your food choices, but there are plenty of vegetables and grains that have multiple different texture possibilities. Common keto recipes often use cucumbers to create tasty fresh sushi wraps and long strips of zucchini or parsnips in place of thick pasta noodles. If you have a hankering for crispy potato chips, but you do not want to sacrifice the calories, carbs, or processed grains, roasting a few large kale leaves in the oven with sea salt, pepper, and vinegar gives you the crunch you want with the nutrients you need. When it comes to substituting whole food groups, you want to remind yourself that the consistent goal is to make all your meals as low in carbohydrates as possible, and as high in fat. Where other diets might encourage you to trim down on your fat intake, the keto diet could always use more fatty acids to fuel your cellular respiration. Avocado oil and sesame seed oil and both fabulous high fat content oils that you can use in your cooking to up the fat content. Keep in mind, however, that both avocado and sesame seed oil have low smoke points, which means they will burn at a lower temperature. Olive oil is a great substitute for canola oil if you want to increase your fat content and keep your oil at a nice high temperature for a good sear. If you enjoy baking, full-fat milk is a great way also to increase your fat content. Both natural, full-fat coconut milk and almond milk will help to up your fat content without also upping your intake of fatty lactose milk sugars and hydrogenated fats. When it comes to flour, there are more carbohydrates in one cup of bleached white flour than you can possibly imagine. Switching out almond flour or hazelnut flour will have the same chemical effect for your baking recipes without harming your ability to reach ketosis.

Keto Diet Sweetening Hacks

Sweetening up your meals and snacks can be one of the most challenging aspects of the keto diet, and if you aren't quite sure how to do so, you might backtrack your ketosis. While we've mentioned Stevia before, a naturally-derived artificial sweetener that comes in liquid, powdered, and granulated forms, there are a few other sweetening tricks that will amp up your keto meals. While you are eating a keto diet, you are going to want to avoid even supposedly "healthy" sweeteners like agave syrup and honey. While honey also comes from bees and is therefore not vegan and often processed, agave is simply incredibly high in sugar content. After Stevia, the next most popular keto sweeteners are Xylitol and Erythritol, also known as "sugar alcohols". Sugar alcohols can be found naturally in small berries, but most of these sweeteners are man-made – which means they can sometimes cause allergies or upset your digestion. It is also worth it to note that sugar alcohols, unlike Stevia, still contain small traces of carbohydrates. Monk fruit sweetener, or monk fruit extract, is the last most popular ketogenic sweetener that you should definitely have in your pantry. Monk fruit sweetener is the holy grail of the keto diet because of its lack of almost any nutritional value – except flavor. Monk fruit extract contains zero carbohydrates, calories, and fat. It also has no sodium, and generally will not affect your digestive processes as much as sugar alcohol. If you do not mind that this sweetener is a bit on the, well, *sweet* side, then monk fruit is the way to go; stick to Stevia if you want zero calories without a sugary aftertaste.

Exercising For Keto Success

Physical fitness on the ketogenic diet is a scientific beast that you will definitely need help in tackling. Remember back to the very first chapter of this book, when we discussed the differences between metabolizing glucose and metabolizing fat. One of these fuel sources can sustain cellular respiration without oxygen, and one of these fuel sources can't. When you are eating a ketogenic diet, you are supplying your body with virtually no daily carbohydrates, which means virtually no glucose. During intense workouts that require your muscle cells to perform anaerobic cellular respiration (which means without oxygen, in case you forgot), you will not have anything to give your hungry body. Without glucose, you will not be able to continue your intense exercise, and you will have to slow down due to intense muscle fatigue. Although this might make it sound like the ketogenic diet is an absolute no-go for athletes who need ample supplies of glucose to perform, that is not the case. As long as you make a few conscious changes to your workout routine and dieting style, you will be able to continue growing your muscles, lifting weights, and performing at your best without compromising your weight loss ketosis. Instead of hitting the gym to perform rep after rep of bicep curls, exercises that work with the keto diet are going to have you closer to the floor than anything.

Keto-friendly exercise routines often focus on strength, stability, flexibility, and sustained low-impact cardio. There is new research that also includes high-intensity interval training as a keto-friendly exercise regime, but we will touch more on that in a bit. For now, you should focus on a new physical fitness routine that includes disciplines like yoga and Pilates. Although these exercises have a minimal impact on your breathing and muscle use, you will still be able to achieve the same toning and strengthening effects that you could with more intense exercises. If you like to stick to activities that focus more on cardio, you will want to make sure that you aren't exerting yourself beyond a certain cardiac threshold. Low impact cardio exercises that work well with a ketogenic lifestyle include running on the elliptical, jogging at a maintainable pace for long periods of time, and biking at a low resistance on a minimal incline percentage. Recent scientific studies have also examined the efficiency of high-intensity interval training in combination with a keto diet, and if you like a workout that presents a challenge, you will be glad to hear the two are relatively compatible.

Keeping Your Gains Going on Keto

For those of you who are worried about giving up your hard-earned muscles and dedicated gym routine just to eat a keto diet, you do not have to be. Luckily, there are plenty of individuals who have tried and tested various methods of fueling intense weight-lifting and athletic training with a keto diet. And the best part is, you will not have to worry about ruining your chance at achieving ketosis. In order to make sure that you are able to grow your muscles, heal your tears, and power through important workouts, you will want to make sure that you tailor your keto diet to give you a boost of carbohydrates before the gym. Though this might sound like risky business, it is entirely manageable as long as you stay organized and on top of your nutrition. Thirty minutes before you work out, athletes on the keto diet recommend that you eat anywhere from twenty-five to fifty grams of carbohydrates. Whether you do this with an energy bar, a meal or snack, or a shake, you should make sure not to increase the amount past fifty grams if you want to maintain ketosis. However, it is important to keep in mind that fifty grams of carbohydrates is quite a lot, and if you are not active enough to justify this amount, you should stick closer to twenty-five in order to maintain your weight loss. If you are planning on working out intensely during your ketogenic reset, make sure you factor in meal prepping extra meals that are heavy in carbohydrates and separate from your keto-friendly high fat entrees. When you are working out strenuously on a keto diet that is already likely to make you weaker than normal, it is incredibly important that you make sure to eat before your workouts (and meal prep your carb doses) so that you do not find yourself skipping a meal to make your training session. Eating on a keto diet is never about compromising on the things that you enjoy, and especially if you enjoy working out in the gym, the keto diet always has room to eat for an athletic lifestyle.

High-Intensity Interval Training

Relatively all of the claims made by the ketogenic diet have been resoundingly approved by the scientific community, but that doesn't mean that we understand quite all of the effects that keto can have on different body types. From what you have learned in these past fitness sections, high-intensity interval training should be a bad idea for keto dieters looking to workout. If you do not have any glucose available for your muscles to catabolize, you are going to be physically unable to move past a certain exertion threshold when your energy runs out. However, there is an interesting quirk to the keto diet and reaching ketosis that fitness experts have recently begun to study more in-depth. This concept would be that of a low-carbohydrate diet like the keto diet actually helping to *improve* intensely, sustained, and fast-moving exercise. Plenty of athletes have recently discovered that, once their bodies reach ketosis, they are able to call forth their old energy levels and perform at the same output in the gym. Even without a fifty-gram carbohydrate load before they begin, many athletes eating keto in full ketosis demonstrate better stamina, a shorter period of recovery, and increased muscle growth when they train with high-intensity intervals on keto. Obviously, fitness and dieting are intimately related, and especially when it comes to such a new and unknown aspect of the keto diet, you should make sure that you are following what your body, and your doctor, say first, before listening to experimental science. That being said, there is no harm in trying out new things, and with so much exciting new research, there is little that can go wrong with simply attempting an exercise routine. Either way, the keto diet will have your back, and there are plenty of other options if high-intensity interval training doesn't quite fit with your ketogenic reset.

Conclusion

Tips for Transitioning Out of a Ketogenic Diet

A ketogenic reset is one of the best healthy eating routines for our modern lifestyles, but even those of us who are won over by the powers of a keto diet will need to transition back to carbohydrates at some point. Keto can absolutely be a life-time eating program, but in order to take care of your body, you should know how to safely ween yourself off of fats, and back onto carbohydrates. Plus, a keto diet is so effective for weight loss. Eventually, you are going to reach your goals – and you might want to be able to eat a donut to celebrate. The ketogenic diet is just as easy to transition out of as it was for you to prepare your body to transition into. And this time, you likely will not experience any of the negative side effects of a carbohydrate flu if you follow the right steps. The key to transitioning off of a keto diet is to try and maintain as many of the healthy habits you learned during keto as possible. Simply tossing away your hard work by re-introducing processed foods, saturated fats, and hydrogenated oils will immediately reverse all of your weight loss results – and have incredibly strenuous effects on your internal organs. Any type of drastic change, like switching *into* keto, has to be taken slowly so as not to shock your body. Remember – glucose is our preferred fuel source, and your body is definitely feeling starved for sugar by the time you are thinking of transitioning out of keto. In order to best maintain the results of your ketosis while also indulging in new food groups, it is time to head back to the grocery store. Like you did when you were preparing your meals, you are going to want to make a plan for what you would like to eat after you leave behind the keto diet. Plan out healthy portions that slowly begin to increase, and decrease, according to normal dietary standards. Off of a keto diet, the recommended macronutrient proportions for the average adult are ten to thirty-five percent proteins, twenty to thirty-five percent fats, and forty-five to sixty-five percent carbohydrates. You will not want to increase your portions to these ratios immediately, but you should slowly grow or shrink to meet them. It is always a good idea, to begin with, the smallest possible amount of carbohydrates before increasing to larger portions. You should also stick to natural, unprocessed, and unbleached grains and carbs that are not filled with sugar when you first reintroduce. Reversing keto is a slow process that normally takes a few weeks. Adding in carbs in minimal amounts to one meal per day is a great plan until your gastrointestinal health returns to normal. If you start to experience a large amount of digestive discomfort while transitioning out of keto, don't worry – your body needs more time to adjust. Cut back on your carbs, keep drinking as much water as possible, and before long, you will be able to work all of your favorite foods back into your diet (in healthier versions of course). While you might also gain some weight and start to feel hungrier than you are used to during ketosis, your transition period should only take two to three weeks to complete, and once you feel comfortable doing so, you are welcome to start to work back towards ketosis if you are tackling the ketogenic reset as a cyclical program.

Final Thoughts

No diet is ever going to be easy, and losing stubborn fat is always going to take more effort than it does to eat junk food. But weight loss does not have to be painful, difficult, and disheartening like so many modern diet trends can make you feel. After reading through this guide, you hopefully understand that the ketogenic reset, and the keto diet in general, is not like any other diet plan you will find on Instagram. When you embark on a ketogenic journey, you are choosing to take a long hard look at what your body truly needs to function at its best. For most of our lives, many of us have listened to nutritionists, doctors, our parents, and the government to make sure that we're eating what we're supposed to. Instead, we should have been taking the time to listen to what our *bodies* were saying, and more importantly – what they *weren't* saying. High levels of obesity, heart disease, bad cholesterol, and diabetes at the end of the twentieth century should have alerted many of us to the harmful processed foods we were eating. But it is far too easy to trust in the opinions of others if you aren't armed with the proper knowledge about your body in the first place. The biological mechanisms that we have been given naturally are perfectly capable of helping us lose weight if we just take the time to understand which tools are required to do so. Once you understand how a ketogenic diet changes your metabolism to consume fats instead of carbohydrates, you can determine what results your body will produce based on the fuel sources that you feed it. Never before has a diet detailed such a circular relationship between our food, our bodies, and our health markers - but that is because a diet has never worked so closely with our natural structures before. When you fuel your body with healthy fats and limited carbohydrates on a keto diet, you can control your body's function and dictate healthier outcomes. Listening to your body's needs and then using natural ingredients to fulfill them is the basic foundation of a ketogenic lifestyle – and it should be the basic foundation of everyone's natural life anyway. Seeking out a ketogenic reset is not just about trying to lose weight or combating difficult medical issues. A ketogenic reset will teach you the value of caring for your body the way your body wants to be cared for, and your biological mechanisms will run better than they ever have as a way of saying "Thank You". If you have enjoyed this instructional manual or found it helpful in any way, please leave a review and let us know. Your journey to achieving a ketogenic reset is the most important thing, and as long as you follow the advice in this guide, you will find that a keto diet can be incredibly easy. Each unique story and insight is invaluable to creating a stronger and more effective ketogenic diet, so be sure to participate in the online community if you start eating keto. We would like to thank you for coming along on this instructional trip, and we wish you the best of luck as you discover the lifetime benefits of the ketogenic reset. Stay safe, stay hydrated, and enjoy what the keto diet can do for you.

198

199

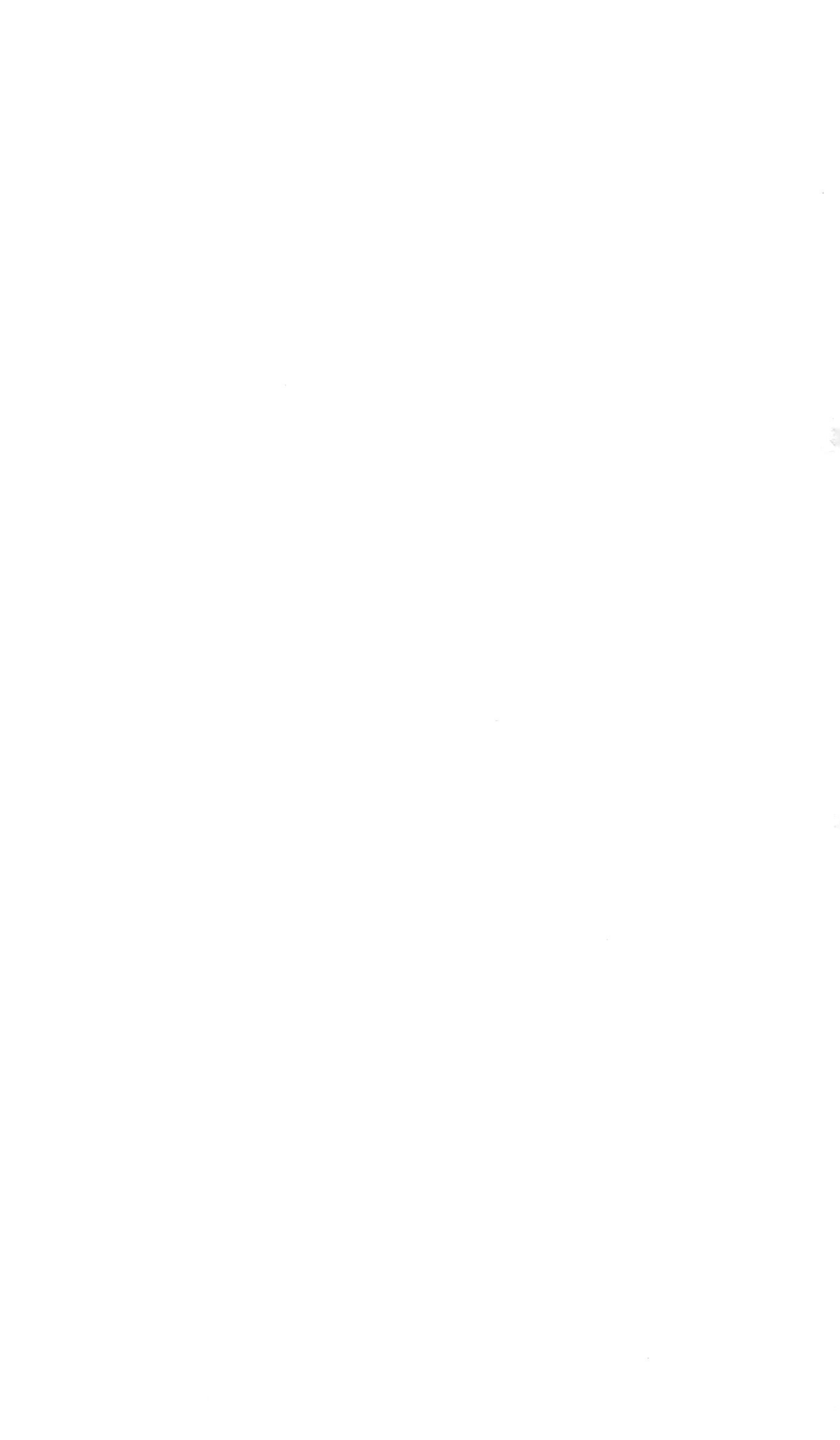

9 781692 383350